God's
Healing Power

I0225247

God's
Healing Power

Karen Henein

GOD'S HEALING POWER
Copyright © 2019 by Karen Henein

All rights reserved. Neither this publication nor any part of this publication may be reproduced or transmitted in any form or by any means, electronic or mechanical, including photocopying, recording or any information storage and retrieval system, without permission in writing from the author.

This material is not intended as a substitution for medical advice. Please consult a physician before undertaking any changes to diet, exercise, or medication.

The content of this publication is based on actual events experienced by the author, described to the author by persons she knows and trusts, or detailed in a biography, autobiography, memoir, book of some other kind, article, or talk presented in a public venue.

Unless otherwise indicated, all scripture quotations are from The Holy Bible, English Standard Version® (ESV®), copyright © 2001 by Crossway, a publishing ministry of Good News Publishers. Used by permission. All rights reserved. Scripture quotations labelled (NIV) are from the Holy Bible, NEW INTERNATIONAL VERSION®, NIV® Copyright © 1973, 1978, 1984, 2011 by Biblica, Inc.® Used by permission. All rights reserved worldwide. Scripture quotations labelled (NLT) are from the Holy Bible, New Living Translation, copyright ©1996, 2004, 2007 by Tyndale House Foundation. Used by permission of Tyndale House Publishers, Inc., Carol Stream, Illinois 60188. All rights reserved. Scripture quotations labelled (NKJV) are from the New King James Version®. Copyright © 1982 by Thomas Nelson, Inc. Used by permission. All rights reserved. Scripture quotations labelled (KJV) are taken from the Holy Bible, King James Version, which is in the public domain.

Some words in scripture verses have been italicized by the author for emphasis.

The Internet addresses and website content referred to herein are accurate at the time of publication (or as of the date specified). They are provided as a resource. The publisher and author do not endorse all of the content on all of websites cited or promise the permanence of such websites or any content contained therein.

ISBN: 978-1-4866-1843-9

Word Alive Press
119 De Baets Street, Winnipeg, MB R2J 3R9
www.wordalivepress.ca

WORD ALIVE
—P R E S S—

Cataloguing in Publication may be obtained through Library and Archives Canada

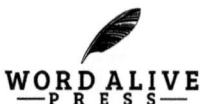

Contents

THANK YOU NOTES

I would like to thank all those who have made this book possible. I received encouragement and support from many family members and friends. Many also prayed for me during the writing process. Thank you!

I thank the advance readers of my manuscript, whose feedback was invaluable: my husband, my son, Reni Horban, Jan Stern, Brenda Hodgson, Patti Town, Jo-anne Lambert, Tanya Clements, and Dawn and Steve Briggs. I also thank those who commented on portions of the manuscript. The knowledge, wisdom, and insights of others have greatly enriched this book.

I am grateful to family members and friends who gave me permission to tell their stories. I trust that their stories will bless and encourage many.

I thank my publisher, Word Alive Press, and those staff members who edited the manuscript, formatted the book, and designed its cover. I am especially grateful to Marina Reis and Kerry Wilson. Thanks also to those who have helped to get the book placed in bricks-and-mortar bookstores and on many electronic platforms.

Above all, I thank God for His help with this book (and every other aspect of my life) and for the lessons, experiences, guidance, and healing He has provided. I hope that God receives great glory for all that He has done.

1

GOD STILL HEALS

Within a four-year span, my son, husband, and father each experienced a life-threatening medical crisis while in their early twenties, late fifties, and early eighties, respectively. My son spent forty days in the hospital, mostly in the Intensive Care Unit (ICU) or the step-down ICU. My husband spent a week in the ICU, and my father slightly less. Each hospitalization was heart wrenching, and each outcome very uncertain at the time. By God's grace and power, all three recovered.

In between the ordeals of my husband and my father (half a year apart), I fought a serious bacterial infection of the bowel, known as C. *difficile*, which I likely acquired while visiting my husband in the hospital. That same year, a close friend suffered a heart attack and underwent triple bypass surgery. I thank God for restoring both my friend and me.

I learned (and relearned) a few things about God's healing power during all those health challenges and while spending hours visiting in hospital rooms, offering recovery support, reviewing what the Bible teaches about healing, and praying for myself and others. I developed greater empathy for the sick and the suffering.

Those incidents are just some of the encounters that I, or a loved one, have had with medical trauma. No doubt you've had your own encounters with illness, injury, surgery, and suffering. Perhaps you've experienced healing.

I once heard a sermon about the importance of sharing our healing stories. Our healing might not be perfect, but any measure of healing is a great gift. If we choose *not* to share our stories, we deprive others of an opportunity to hear about God's healing power. That sermon encouraged me to write about some healing stories, alongside a discussion of what I believe the Bible teaches about God's healing power.

Asaph (King David's music director) instructed God's people to "… tell to the coming generation the glorious deeds of the Lord, and his might, and the wonders that he has done" (Psalm 78:4). King David did just that. He had been sick and had cried out to God. He had prayed: "Be gracious to me, O Lord, for I am languishing; heal me, O Lord, for my bones are troubled" (Psalm 6:2). After being healed, David wrote: "Praise the Lord, my soul; all my inmost being, praise his holy name. Praise the Lord, my soul, and forget not all his benefits—who forgives all your sins and heals all your diseases" (Psalm 103:1–3, NIV). David also wrote: "I will give thanks to the Lord with my whole heart; I will recount all of your wonderful deeds" (Psalm 9:1).

God has healed me many times. He has healed many people I know. I, too, want to recount His awesome deeds.

As you read this book, I hope you remember your own stories of how God has healed you or your loved ones. I also hope that you reflect on what God has already taught you from His Word on the topic of healing.

Perhaps your story is still in progress. You might be suffering greatly. Maybe you're dealing with a death sentence some doctor has delivered, or maybe you feel you've been given a life sentence because you struggle with a chronic disease. *Is healing possible for me?* you wonder.

Perhaps you know stories that didn't turn out as positively as you had hoped, and you're full of questions about the scope of God's healing power or His inclination to heal. Perhaps a loved one has died.

Please don't put this book down. You are not alone. I had a miscarriage after experiencing bleeding during my second pregnancy. Many prayers did not result in that little life being saved. A few close friends have lost their husbands to cancer in recent years. I've known many other people of great faith who trusted God for healing yet still died before reaching old age.

We must address the troubling reality that some faithful, faith-filled, praying, and prayed-for loved ones die before we want them to. Why God allows seemingly untimely deaths will remain, in part, a mystery to us. To gain *some* insight into God's perspective on this, we'll consider biblical verses dealing with lifespan, death, and life after death. The reality of death—which each one must face at some age—should not deter us from seeking God's power to heal us while we're still alive.

A Childhood Experience

I first developed an interest in God's power to heal when I was nine years young. During that difficult year, I was struck by an unusual affliction that took many doctors months to figure out. Over the winter and spring, my muscles progressively weakened. At first, I just felt strangely tired after my school day. Then my winter coat seemed unduly heavy on sagging shoulders. Eventually, the weight of it became almost unbearable. Raising my arm to comb my hair took herculean effort. The time came when I couldn't finish tests at school because I didn't have the strength to push my pencil for half an hour.

Before that onset of weakness, I had been an active kid. I turned cartwheel after cartwheel on the lawn in summer and tobogganed for hours in the winter. During school recesses, I played football with the boys, skipped rope with the girls, or enjoyed a lively game of tag with whoever else joined in. I'd bet I could run as fast as a purse-snatching street thief back in those days. The debilitating muscle fatigue cruelly invaded an energetic life.

I stayed in the hospital twice that year for a total of five weeks.

During the first hospital admission, the doctors ran tests, consulted together, and concluded there was nothing wrong with me. Perhaps, they said, I just needed more exercise to overcome my muscle weakness. They sent me home, and I began a nightly regimen of skipping with a jump rope. Even a few minutes of such exercise made me feel like an Olympic athlete might feel after a marathon training session. Despite my efforts, I grew even weaker.

Then one day, after sitting on the gym floor for a school assembly, I couldn't stand up again to head back to class. My teacher phoned my parents, who phoned my pediatrician. He put me back in the hospital.

During my second hospital stay, after another week of tests and being the subject of a grand-rounds assembly of doctors from across the continent, I finally received a diagnosis. I had an autoimmune disease called juvenile dermatomyositis (JDM), a kind of inflammatory muscle disease. Back in the 1960s, that particular disease hadn't yet been the subject of much medical study. It was no wonder it had taken a while for the doctors to figure out what was wrong with me. They were finally tipped off by the development of a unique skin rash (which accounts for the "dermato" prefix).

JDM is quite rare. About three per every million children in the United States and Canada are diagnosed with the disease each year. In the 1960s, Toronto had a population of about two million people of all ages. The number of children would have been much less than that. It's possible that I was the only child diagnosed with JDM in Toronto that year.

After the diagnosis, more doctors came to see me. Sometimes I had to show large groups of gaping doctors what I could and couldn't do with various muscles. I remember shivering in a skimpy hospital gown while I was put through my paces in a packed hospital amphitheatre. I now realize that my moments of excruciating embarrassment and physical discomfort in that crowded room probably contributed to the medical literature and might have later benefitted other children suffering with JDM.

The attention scared me. Even at the age of nine, I could surmise that the interest of so many doctors in my case meant that I was suffering from a serious disease.

In the early days of my second hospitalization, I was too weak to walk or even stand. Nurses took turns pushing me around the ward while I sat passively in a wheelchair. I couldn't push the wheels around on my own. I don't know if electric wheelchairs had been invented by that time, but I know they didn't exist in my pediatric ward. When I went for tests on other hospital floors, I had to be strapped to a gurney. Watching the ceiling tiles whiz by overhead, en route to yet another unfamiliar room, made my little heart thump wildly.

Much of the time, I was confined to my bed, and the days passed slowly. Thankfully, I had a window in my room. Sometimes a nurse would help me get seated in a chair beside the window. I could then see the busy avenue below and the gorgeous trees, bushes, and flowers growing in the boulevard between the traffic lanes. I marvelled at the beauty of spring as it unfolded before me. God was out there.

At night, I sometimes stared at my face in the mirror. I accessed that miserable mirror by flipping up the top of the narrow portable table that could be wheeled into place over my bed. I barely recognized myself. The high-dose corticosteroid pills I swallowed a few times a day had produced rosy chipmunk cheeks. That was the least serious, but most noticeable, side effect of the potent medication. I wondered why the same God who made the beautiful springtime blossoms outside was allowing me to languish in the hospital with a body that failed me and crushed my spirit.

I spent long hours alone. My siblings weren't allowed to visit me because of the draconian hospital rules of that era. My parents could only come during strict visiting hours. They had a long drive from the suburbs into the city, so they couldn't visit often.

I had few other visitors during my weeks in the hospital. Perhaps that's one reason that I have such a clear memory of my Uncle Phil and Pastor Kenn coming to visit me one day. They spent a while praying for me out loud. I felt comforted by their long conversation with God.

They talked like they knew Him well and seemed quite sure He was listening. I didn't understand all of their words, but I *did* grasp that they were fervently petitioning God to restore my health. I had such a sense of peace and calm during and after that prayer. God's presence filled the room. He was no longer just in the gardens outside my window. I felt a gentle stirring of hope deep within.

I didn't get better instantly. It mattered to me, however, that two men of obvious faith had spoken aloud to God and told Him all about me. I waited with great interest to see what God was going to do. Did God really care about a little girl trapped in a hospital bed by muscles in mutiny? I dared to faintly believe that He did, with a faith as weak as my muscles.

Nurses continued to roll me around the pediatric ward on my little silver-wheeled chariot. I suffered from great angst about whether I would ever be able to walk again. I don't remember a single doctor or nurse talking to me about when—or if—I would recover strength or mobility. My pediatrician came to my bedside daily. He didn't tell me anything about my condition or prognosis, but at least he seemed to care.

My strength began to return, little by little. The delightful day came when I could get out of bed with minimal assistance. I could then hobble over to the chair by the window by myself. Eventually, I could slowly shuffle a short distance down the hall to the kids' playroom. It took every particle of my strength and energy to do that, but it was worth it. I enjoyed talking with other kids, even those a lot younger than me. It felt quite peculiar, at the age of nine, to be playing blocks with preschoolers some mornings, but the company of others was always welcome.

Later that spring, I returned home and back to school. Still too weak to play with the other kids, I sat silently on some cement steps at recess and watched my classmates frolic. My former friends didn't know what to say, so they generally avoided me. I felt abandoned. I was too tired to chum with others after school. Television and books became my best friends.

I went to summer camp that year. I was sad that I could barely play dodgeball or baseball. The hike I was forced to take felt like it would be the end of me. My best camp experience involved participating in a "church" service in the forest. We sat on horizontal log benches, arranged in a circle, in a cathedral of vibrant green trees. Sunlight streamed down through the branches. God felt so present again. I sensed His encouragement.

Although my ongoing recovery wasn't nearly fast enough for my liking, I *did* recognize that, over the months, I had improved significantly since that pivotal day when my uncle and my pastor prayed for me.

I prayed as best as I could on my own. My prayers were probably along the lines of: "Please, God, make me better. Make my life normal again. Make this all end like some bad dream I can wake up from. Amen." My faith was that of a child, as simple as faith can get. I had no awareness then of the intense spiritual battle others waged on my behalf.

The following school year, I could play sports again, but not very well. For some JDM kids, it can take years to rebuild functional muscle strength. I spent about two years redeveloping my muscle strength (which never fully returned to the "old normal"). I avoided team sports as much as I could, because I was afraid of letting my teammates down. When captains were assigned to pick teams in gym class, I was always the last person selected. Later, during my teen years, I gravitated toward skating and singles tennis, because no one else had to depend on my limited athletic prowess. The main thing I did on my own time was walk. I became obsessed with walking, an activity I still love.

Although doctors and medication played their important roles, I ultimately credit God with the eventual demise of my childhood disease. To God belongs the greatest glory. I thank Him that the disabling disease I struggled with is now ancient history.

The autoimmune disease could have become a chronic condition, lasting a lifetime. I could have cycled in and out of active disease,

disability, treatment, and remission. I might have experienced significant and lasting muscle atrophy or contracture. JDM could also have
affected other parts of my body, such as my lungs, and could have
been complicated by secondary conditions, such as arthritis. Medications with brutal side effects might have become my lot.

I thank God that, by His power, grace, and mercy, I have been
in steady remission for more than half a century. Perhaps I've been
permanently healed. I choose to believe that.

During more than four-and-a-half decades of adult life, I have
been strong. Strong enough. No, this story doesn't end with me win-
ning an Olympic medal, but God has given me much opportunity to
walk, far and wide. My nine-year-old self, trapped in a bed, a wheelchair, or a chair, could never have imagined where my legs would
one day carry me. Even though I only spent weeks in a wheelchair, it
was long enough to make me *forever* grateful for the simple ability to
walk. I can testify that God gives "… power to the faint, and to him
who has no might he increases strength" (Isaiah 40:29). I *never* take
my measure of health, strength, and energy for granted. I often thank
God for these gifts. In my sixties, I'm still walking all over the place
(although some days my knees or hips complain). I continue to rejoice
in my level of mobility.

I wish I had the power to make every reader healthy and strong.
I don't. But I can talk to you about the one who *does* have the power
to heal. And I can pray that He heals you and heals those you love. I
pause to pray, at this moment, for every single person who ever reads
this book and for the ailing people they care about.

Ever since God healed my childhood affliction, I have not doubt-
ed that God exists, that He rules the universe with power, and that He
is a loving God. Along the way, I have fully committed my life to Him,
and I have acquired even firmer faith that He can heal.

After my childhood illness, I developed special sympathy for
family members or friends when health problems weakened them.
I've been quick to pray for them. I've paid keen attention to when and
how God healed them, especially those who sustained grave injuries,

underwent major surgeries, or battled serious illnesses. So many of them have been healed.

We have *all* received *some* measure of healing over our lifetimes, have we not? If you're old enough to be reading this, you've likely been healed several times. I make a safe bet that you fell down on the ground when you were a child and scraped your knees. (Maybe, like me, you still sometimes fall down and scrape your knees.) You might have bled, maybe a lot, but the bleeding stopped and the cuts scabbed over. Eventually, the scabbing fell away and fresh new skin reappeared. I venture to guess that you have battled colds, flues, headaches, and sore throats. I suspect that those afflictions vanished, often without medical aid. Stop to think of the miraculous fact that our bodies have been preprogrammed by God to heal themselves when such health challenges occur.

Have you ever cut your finger or twisted an ankle? Have you had to rush to the toilet with a gastrointestinal bug of some kind? Did those maladies come to an end one day? Who healed you? Beyond the bandages you applied, the pills you swallowed, and whatever doctors you consulted, who ultimately healed you?

Most of us have been healed multiple times. We've recovered from minor medical ailments and, perhaps, from major issues. Although all of us will die at some point of one thing or another, that reality doesn't negate the fact that God has sustained our lives up until now. He has already granted us *some* measure of health and offered *some* measure of healing for *some* period of time.

Later, when we exit this temporal world, scripture promises that we will receive a new body that we can enjoy for all eternity. Every believer will receive that miracle.

What We Will Explore Together

Many Bible verses discuss healing. This book will present over seven hundred verses, mined from the book of Genesis right through to the book of Revelation, related to healing. As you meditate on this rich array, you can form your own viewpoint regarding what you believe the Bible teaches about God's healing power. You don't have to agree with every word I write. I don't pretend to fully understand everything the Bible says about healing. I'll be pleased if your main focus as you read is on discerning for yourself what God has said about healing.

Here are some highlights of what I've come to believe. Healing from God flows from:

- His unlimited power
- His character (including attributes such as His love, kindness, compassion, empathy, mercy, and grace)
- His nature as the generous giver of good gifts, including the gifts of life, health, and eternal life
- His benevolent volition (His expressed covenant and desire to heal His people)
- His all-surpassing glory

I've also learned, over the years, that we have our own part to play in our healing stories. We can partner with God in the healing process. His power to heal flows *to* us and *through* us (and *to* our ailing loved ones) in a variety of ways that involve our active participation. I encourage you to learn about those ways and to put them into practice. It's important that we understand the dynamics of healing. Let's consider what part God plays in the process and what He expects us to do.

Those who prayed for me as a child knew much about all of this. I prayed with the faith of a child. They prayed with a more mature, knowledge-based, experience-affirmed faith. (Of course, both kinds of faith are of great value in God's eyes.)

How does God's healing power flow to us and through us? His healing power flows through:

- our personal relationship with Him
- our efforts to take care of our physical, mental, and emotional health

- our knowledge of God's Word and reliance upon it
- faith, trust, and hope
- prayer
- gratitude and praise
- obedience to God
- reverent use of the name of Jesus
- full recognition of what was accomplished on the cross
- the Spirit, who dwells within believers
- our acting on the authority we have been granted as His followers
- our patience and perseverance in partnering with God in all of this

God can also bless our efforts to seek practical help from doctors and other healthcare professionals. It might be necessary to take medication or undergo surgery. I don't want to discourage anyone from seeking medical help. On the contrary, I strongly encourage everyone to diligently seek appropriate medical care.

Our support networks can also greatly help us in the recovery process.

Can you imagine the *combined* power of everything I've just described? God's power can flow mightily in us, through us, and through others in all the ways I've mentioned. The cumulative effect can be quite astonishing.

The timing and the method of healing are in God's control. God could allow us to first go through one or more seasons of suffering. As we wait for healing, we can search for any obstacles that might be blocking God's healing power.

I look around me and see that the need for healing is great. Despite all of its wondrous advancements, medical science cannot heal every person of every ailment. Thankfully, God's power to heal extends far beyond the reach of human medical care.

We might get sick, we might get injured, and we might need surgery. Our loved ones will also likely encounter such setbacks. But with

God's power in play, we can press on to the other side of such health challenges (or, at least, be able to minimize and manage them) for as long as God grants us life and breath.

THE NATURE OF OUR HEALING GOD

2

GOD'S POWER

Our God is powerful. All powerful. His power is superlative, supreme, infinite, and eternal.

God reigns sovereign over everyone and everything. Almighty God can do anything. Jesus proclaimed: "For nothing will be impossible with God" (Luke 1:37). Jesus also declared: "... with God all things are possible" (Matthew 19:26).

God has the power to heal our bodies. He can heal every sickness, disease, and injury. Jesus, the Son of God, displayed that power when He walked this earth.

Matthew 4:23 testifies: "... he [Jesus] went throughout all Galilee, teaching in their synagogues and proclaiming the gospel of the kingdom and healing every disease and every affliction among the people."

Matthew 9:35 further reports: "And Jesus went throughout all the cities and villages…healing every disease and every affliction."

Matthew 12:15b simply states: "... many followed him, and he healed them all…"

Matthew 15:30–31 specifies:

... great crowds came to him [Jesus], bringing with them the lame,
the blind, the crippled, the mute, and many others, and they put
them at his feet, and he healed them, so that the crowd wondered,
when they saw the mute speaking, the crippled healthy, the lame
walking, and the blind seeing...

Luke affirmed that Jesus healed a wide range of physical ailments: "... when the sun was setting, all those who had any who were sick with various diseases brought them to him, and he laid his hands on every one of them and healed them" (Luke 4:40). The Gospel of Luke goes on to describe many healings on further occasions.

No ailment exists beyond the scope of God's healing power. Not paralysis or blindness, not deafness or brain seizures. Not cancer, heart disease, or any autoimmune conditions. No sickness is too serious, too advanced, or too rare. God can heal anything and everything. Nothing is too hard for Him.

You might be struggling to accept such a sweeping proposition. Perhaps you're thinking about someone who died without being fully healed, or someone who has been sick for a long time. Perhaps you're discouraged by an illness that keeps returning to you. I understand what huge mental roadblocks those situations can create. We will consider those roadblocks in later chapters.

This present chapter is not about why God allows some people to die before their old age, or why He allows them to die at any age while still in a state of sickness, or why He allows anyone to suffer. I'm simply trying to establish that God *does* have the power to heal any physical condition. This chapter is about God possessing that power, not His exercise of that power. We'll have opportunity later to consider the basis upon which He exercises His healing power. We know that He doesn't always exercise that power.

Let's invest a few moments in taking a broader look at God's overall power.

God's Creative Power

Let's begin by considering God's *creative* power. The book of Genesis describes how God created the entire universe. I believe He did. I don't buy into the murky theory that everything somehow came into existence from some mysterious chemical soup that existed in the universe at the beginning of time. Who made the soup? If there was a Big Bang way back when, who initiated it? And why? I find scientific explanations about the origin of our universe that leave God out of the picture to be wholly unsatisfying, both intellectually and spiritually.

God created the galaxies, planets, stars, sun, and moon. He made the earth and its oceans, continents, mountains, deserts, forests, lakes, and rivers. He added animals, fish, birds, insects, grass, and flowers. Looking around our world convinces me that an all-powerful being (of infinitely higher intelligence than humankind possesses) must surely have created the beautiful, complex, diverse realm of nature.

Some choose to be wilfully blind to the open display of God's power in nature. Romans 1:18–20 asserts:

> *For the wrath of God is revealed from heaven against all ungodliness and unrighteousness of men, who by their unrighteousness suppress the truth. For what can be known about God is plain to them, because God has shown it to them. For his invisible attributes, namely, his eternal power and divine nature, have been clearly perceived, ever since the creation of the world, in the things that have been made. So they are without excuse.*

God created humankind. He created you and me. Psalm 139:13–15 tells us that He formed us in our mothers' wombs and that His creation of us is wonderful. God invented the idea of you and me a long time ago. He created us to match the custom designs He had in mind. God gave to each one of us the precious gift of life on this earth. I wouldn't be writing this, and you wouldn't be reading it, but for that gift.

Our God-created physical bodies are indeed *amazing*.

Our bodies each contain about ten *octillion* atoms. (Add twenty-seven zeros after the number "ten" to appreciate how big a number that is.) One human body contains more atoms than the estimated number of stars in the universe. Ninety percent of those atoms are replaced each year. In fact, every hour about one trillion trillion atoms get replaced in your body and mine. (That double trillion is not a typo!) That's a lot of ongoing creation! We conduct our daily business without being conscious of that constant creative process.[1]

We each have more than eighteen billion trillion air molecules in our lungs. We breathe around 23,000 times every day. Every twenty-four hours, our hearts contract about 100,000 times. That amounts to billions of heartbeats in the average lifetime. We each have billions of red blood cells that carry oxygen to our tissues. Each body creates more than two million new red blood cells per second. About fifty billion white blood cells in each body fight billions of harmful microbes (such as bad bacteria and viruses). Each human brain has at least ten billion neurons. Every neuron connects with thousands of other neurons, establishing about one hundred trillion interconnections in a single brain.[2]

Such facts demonstrate God's extraordinary design of our bodies. They have been made with brilliant precision, exquisite form, fantastic function, and genius dynamics beyond our full comprehension. They bear striking evidence of God's creative nature.

If you don't believe that God, by His mighty power, created our world and your own breathing being, then you'll likely have difficulty believing in His power to heal.

If you, like me, *do* believe that God created this entire universe and each marvellously made human being in it, then you're primed to believe He can heal what He made in the first place. When you pray for healing, I invite you to pause, for even a moment, to ponder the enormity of God's creation. Then believe that the same God who has the power to create has the power to heal. Like the psalmist, we can say: "I lift up my eyes to the hills. From where does my help come? My help comes from the Lord, who made heaven and earth" (Psalm 121:1–2).

God's Sustaining Power

God also has *sustaining* power. He can sustain whatever He has created for as long as He wants to sustain it. He's the gracious sustainer of your life and mine.

I invite you to appreciate your physical body, however imperfect it might presently be. Life is still surging through you. You might be experiencing problems with your body, and might require medical aid, but your heart still beats and your lungs still breathe. Your brain remains capable of processing these words. God has chosen to sustain your life until this moment in time.

If you're concerned about the medical condition of a loved one, thank God that He has sustained *their* life until this moment, too. Where there is life, there can be hope.

I had several days to focus on (and plead for) God's sustaining power during a health crisis in my family. My husband, Sam, was hospitalized for a major intracerebral hemorrhage. I had taken him to the local emergency department after he complained that he was experiencing the worst headache of his life. After Sam was transferred to the Intensive Care Unit (ICU), one of his doctors explained Sam's medical condition. In the hollow space in the centre of Sam's brain (that should normally just be filled with cerebrospinal fluid), a massive amount of blood had pooled because of a burst blood vessel in the brain. The hollow space wasn't large enough to contain the cerebrospinal fluid and such a large amount of blood. The space was being forced to expand, putting pressure on the surrounding brain tissue. The brain tissue couldn't be pushed outwards much more, because the tissue was encased inside the bone of Sam's skull. If the volume of blood continued to increase, Sam would need immediate brain surgery. A team of neurosurgeons was already on standby at another hospital.

I knew from the outset of his diagnosis that Sam was at significant risk of death. (I have since read that, for Sam's kind of spontaneous brain hemorrhage, the death rate is 34–50 percent within thirty days after onset, with half of those deaths occurring in the first two days.)

I also knew that even if Sam lived, he was at risk of brain damage from blood seeping into the brain tissue. Cognitive abilities, such as comprehension and communication, could be compromised.

The "brain bleed" brought bad enough news. One ICU doctor then reported that Sam was in stage-four heart failure. Further, his kidneys weren't functioning properly. Sam could go into renal failure. His whole body could shut down. The doctor (who knew Sam personally) had tears staining his cheeks as he relayed this news. He humbly admitted his team had very limited control over what would transpire.

The situation seemed hopeless. How much I needed God's power to come down! I appealed to Him to sustain Sam's life. I prayed every moment I could and activated a large number of trusty prayer warriors. Despite all the bleak news, I thanked God for sustaining Sam from one moment to the next.

Sam remained in the ICU for a week and then spent another week in an upstairs ward. Early on, Sam couldn't stay awake or speak for very long. When he did speak, his words often made no sense. As if a television channel was being changed, Sam went from being present in a conversation and appropriate in his responses, to saying confused and even ludicrous things. At one point, he barely had the strength to whisper words in my ear, and I couldn't make out what he was trying to say.

At least the medical staff could rouse Sam on demand for one minute of every hour during each twenty-four-hour cycle. Simply opening his eyes or making any noise after a nurse shook his body counted as being roused. If at any point Sam failed to rouse, he would be rushed to neurosurgery. After a few days of such monitoring, the doctors determined that the brain bleed had been brought under enough control that surgery wouldn't be necessary.

I kept thanking God for sustaining my husband. During the critical early days, when Sam's life flickered like a lamp in a power brownout, I knew God Almighty could prevent a total blackout. I further reckoned that if God could sustain Sam through the acute phase of a major brain bleed, He could also eventually heal Sam's brain, heart, and kidneys. That brain bleed happened more than six years ago. God has sustained Sam's life right up to this moment and has granted significant healing.

If you're going through a medical ordeal, I invite you to thank God that He has sustained you (or your loved one) up to this very hour. And then choose to believe: The God who is powerful enough to sustain our lives surely has the power to heal us. I encourage you to stop focusing on the power of disease or dysfunction and focus instead on the power of God.

God's Transformative Power

God also has *transformative* power. He can change things. All of creation is subject to change. We can see that every day as morning turns into afternoon, then evening into nightfall. Liquid water can turn into steam or ice. Crashing waves can wear down a sea cliff, transforming a solid rockface into tiny pebbles and sand.

We are constantly changing, too. Sometimes we initiate the changes. Other times, God changes us. God can transform us spiritually. God can also transform us physically. If our bodies are diseased or injured, He can change them. God not only creates, He recreates. He renews. He restores. If God created our brains, eyes, ears, bones, skin, muscles, and joints (indeed, *every* part of our bodies), can He not repair them?

We mentioned earlier that trillions of our cells turn over every day. God *routinely* replaces diseased, dysfunctional, or injured cells with new, healthy cells. Every few days, for example, all of the cells that line our intestinal tracts change over. Our skin cells get replaced every few weeks without us even thinking about it. At this very moment, cellular change is occurring in your body and mine.

Other changes routinely occur. When harmful bacteria invade the gut, they typically get chased down through bowel and bladder and eliminated from our bodies. When blood pressure rises in an adrenaline-fuelled moment, it usually returns to normal once the stressor disappears. As we sleep, miniscule tears in our muscles get mended.

Such things happen regularly while we work through our days and sleep through our nights. God recreates, renews, and restores our bodies in ways we take for granted.

Other times, we're more consciously aware of God's power to renew and restore. We skin our knees when we fall down. Flesh is damaged. It might become inflamed, maybe even infected. Perhaps it will bleed, sting, or throb. Over time, new skin replaces the damaged layer of skin. Our leg might get bruised when we bump into something. The bruise turns various colours over the following days and then eventually disappears. These are examples of God's transformative, restorative power in action. All of our body organs, cells, and systems have some measure of built-in resilience.

God has the power to transform our bodies, no matter what condition they're in, no matter how serious the physical irregularity appears to be. Disease or injury transforms our bodies in *de*structive ways. God can *re*construct our bodies and their systems. Pastor A. B. Simpson once wrote that when God heals, sometimes "demolition" precedes "renovation."[3]

I chose to believe in God's transformative power while Sam slowly recovered from the brain bleed. At first, Sam couldn't eat and didn't want to eat. Fluids hydrated him intravenously. Verbal responses kept wavering. For days, he languished in bed. I chose to believe that Sam would eat, drink, speak normally, and walk again. When I wondered if he would ever again feed himself, bathe himself, dress himself, drive, or work as a doctor, I had to consciously immerse my thoughts in what I knew about God's transformative power. I kept reassuring my faltering heart: God can transform; God can transform; God can transform. He had transformed me from a weak, sick little nine-year-old girl who couldn't walk, into a woman who twice spent full years backpacking across continents.

All physical processes are programmed to be dynamic, not static. Transformation happens one nanosecond at a time. Watch a hospital monitor and you can see how pulse, heart rhythm, and blood pressure can change from moment to moment. Transformation might happen invisibly for a while. It might take some time to fully perceive it.

Over days, Sam began sipping water again. At first, he could only press his lips against a water-soaked, pink sponge. When he started eating, I spoon-fed him soup and Jell-O for a while. His words slowly made better sense. By week's end, he could hobble over to the bathroom with a nurse bracing his arm. Then the day came when he ventured into the corridor with a walker.

By the next week, Sam could feed himself and shower. He began walking around the ward at my side. One doctor friend marvelled at how far Sam had bounced back from the brink of either death or disaster.

An MRI at the six-week point showed that the cerebral hemorrhaging had stopped. The mass of accumulated blood in the brain was clearing. Thankfully, the MRI also revealed that there was no brain tumour, a possibility that had not been ruled out until then.

A few months passed before Sam could go back to work for even a few hours a day. It took yet further months before he could work longer hours.

God doesn't always transform us back to our former state. We cannot expect to be fully the same after serious sickness, injury, or surgery. Only one healing story in the entire Bible refers to a complete or perfect healing (Acts 3:16). I sometimes wonder if the healing of others (in Bible accounts) wasn't always absolute, although I imagine that each healing was likely very substantial. In our time, God often gives a great measure of healing but not necessarily perfect healing. God doesn't give everyone a perfect body to begin with, so why do we expect perfect healing? Nothing is perfect in this fallen world.

God didn't fully restore me to my former self after my childhood struggle with JDM. My arm muscles were damaged more than my other muscles. No matter how much I exercise those arm muscles, they will only strengthen to a certain degree. I can thankfully perform most everyday tasks. That level of strength is all I need. I'm not too shy to ask for help if I have trouble opening a jar. God didn't heal me perfectly, but He gave me a very great measure of healing. God also gave Sam a great measure of healing after the brain bleed.

Isaiah 40:30–31 declares:

> *Even youths shall faint and be weary, and young men shall fall exhausted; but they who wait for the Lord shall renew their strength; they shall mount up with wings like eagles; they shall run and not be weary; they shall walk and not faint.*

It's our testimony that God provided both Sam and me with renewed strength, energy, and ability to function reasonably well in our everyday lives. God *can* transform the weak into the strong. We are living proof.

Aside from our health challenges, we are all slowly aging. Aging is a form of continuous transformation, and most of it isn't in a positive direction. God designed the aging process. We must accept that. We cannot expect to be the same at sixty years old as we were at twenty. We can still seek *some* positive transformation as we age. It's never too late to exercise more and eat better and become a stronger version of ourselves, with God's help. Realistically, though, we know that the aging body will experience some measure of deterioration.

But we can be of good cheer. God saves the best for last. Our eternal transformation will gift us with *perfect* indestructible bodies.

God's Resurrection Power

God also has *resurrection* power. God can bring the dead back to life. This power astounds me more than His creative, sustaining, and transformative power. The Bible provides several examples of God's resurrection power.

Matthew 9:18–25 tells the story of a synagogue leader who approached Jesus and entreated: "My daughter has just died, but come and lay your hand on her, and she will live" (v. 18). Moved by such faith, Jesus followed the man to his home. Jesus told the crowd gathered there that the man's daughter was not dead, just sleeping. They laughed at Him. They knew what death looked like. The girl had probably stopped breathing and lost her pulse. Her face had likely frozen into the rigid mask of death. Perhaps her whole body had already become cold and stiff. Undaunted by the laughter, Jesus took the girl by the hand, and she rose up.

Mark 5:21–42 captures another remarkable story. A man named Jairus came to Jesus. Falling on his knees, Jairus pleaded for the healing of his dying daughter. He begged Jesus to come back to his home to lay His hands on his little girl. Some men arrived and announced that it was too late. The little girl was already dead. Jesus wasn't deterred. Instead, He turned to Jairus and told him: "Don't be afraid; just believe" (Mark 5:36b, NIV). Five powerful words.

Jesus then went to the home of Jairus, where He encountered much wailing and crying. In Middle Eastern culture, people often outwardly and dramatically express their grief. The young girl must have been unmistakeably dead.

Only Jesus (and perhaps Jairus, if he had embraced His challenge to believe) refused to accept the situation. Jesus walked into the home, approached the body of the little girl, took her by the hand, and told her to get up. She did rise up. We can only imagine the looks on the faces of the distraught family and friends in that home.

In Luke 7:12–15, we can read yet another amazing story:

> *As he [Jesus] drew near to the gate of the town, behold, a man who had died was being carried out, the only son of his mother, and she was a widow, and a considerable crowd from the town was with her. And when the Lord saw her, he had compassion on her and said to her, "Do not weep." Then he [Jesus] came up and touched the bier, and the bearers stood still. And he said, "Young man, I say to you, arise." And the dead man sat up and began to speak, and Jesus gave him to his mother.*

Then there is the spectacular story of Lazarus, recorded at John 11:1–44. This story stands out because Lazarus had already been dead a few *days*, sealed in an airless tomb, before Jesus brought him back to life.

Jesus is, of course, *the* most important person resurrected from the dead by God's mighty power. Jesus has been resurrected permanently. He will never have to taste death again (as the two young girls, the widow's son, and Lazarus eventually had to).

If you haven't read about the resurrection of Jesus, I encourage you to read the four gospel accounts in Matthew 28, Mark 16, Luke 24, and John 20 and 21. The resurrection of Jesus is the most glorious story ever told.

Years ago, I read *Evidence that Demands a Verdict* by Josh McDowell.[4] As a trial lawyer, I was trained and experienced in the art of critically reviewing all evidence pertaining to a particular event and then considering, on the preponderance of evidence, what most likely happened. I respected McDowell's detailed presentation of the evidence regarding various biblical events. He examined the records of the death and resurrection of Jesus. McDowell considered the four gospel accounts but also referred to accounts written at the time by Jewish and Roman authors. He concluded that the resurrection of Jesus is historical fact. Like McDowell, I am thoroughly convinced that the resurrection of Jesus did occur. The documentary evidence (both in the Bible and beyond) weighs heavily in favour of this. Jesus appeared in bodily form to more than five hundred witnesses on multiple occasions after His crucifixion, His burial, and the discovery of the empty tomb. (In a modern court, it's acceptable to have only one or two witnesses to testify about some event.)

If you have any doubts about the resurrection of Jesus, I invite you to explore the biblical accounts and the broader historical record. Settle your mind on this issue. Ask the risen Christ to reveal Himself to you.

Jesus promises that *we* will be resurrected too, one day, if we believe in Him as the living Son of God. Those who have entered into a personal relationship with God, based on what Jesus accomplished on the cross, can look forward to eternal life: "For God so loved the world, that he gave his only Son, that whoever believes in him should not perish but have eternal life" (John 3:16). This astonishing promise is mentioned throughout the New Testament.

This is fantastic news. Most of us will receive God's healing touch throughout our lives many times over. But at some point, our life on this earth *will* end. Our bodies *will* perish. Believers need not dread this. Our redeemed spirits will live on forever, and our old bodies will be resurrected and recreated into imperishable bodies that will also last forever. That comforted me during the days I thought I might lose my husband after his brain bleed.

Does your health problem seem a little smaller now that you've thought about God's resurrection power? If He can raise the dead, He can certainly heal a broken leg, a concussion, an infection, or even cancer.

Our All-Powerful God

Now that we have stepped back to broadly ponder our all-powerful God, we can better believe in His specific power to heal those He created. When you pray for healing, I encourage you to remember the boundless spectrum of God's incomparable power.

3

GOD'S CHARACTER

For years, I focused my faith on God's *power* to heal. I later learned to also consider His character qualities. I presently appeal to Him for healing on the basis of both His character and His power.

We can acquire greater faith and boldness in praying for healing as we grow in our appreciation of God's marvellous attributes and understand *why* He is motivated to heal. In this chapter, we will examine a few of His traits.

Love

According to 1 John 4:8, God is love. His being radiates love like sunshine radiates warmth and light if we step out of the shadows into it.

God's love is perfect and constant. It never fails. It will never end.

Nothing can separate us from God's love. God will not abandon us or forget about us. He loves us continuously. King David exclaimed: "How precious is your steadfast love, O God!" (Psalm 36:7a).

The apostle Paul wrote: "… I pray that you, being rooted and established in love, may have power… to grasp how wide and long and high and deep is the love of Christ…" (Ephesians 3:17–18, NIV). Paul later scribed: "May the Lord direct your hearts to the love of God and to the steadfastness of Christ" (2 Thessalonians 3:5). God loves *you*.

If you're a parent, consider how much you love your children. When they're sick, you'll likely do anything you can to help them feel better. You'll let them stay home from school. You'll put your work plans on the back burner (as much as possible) so that you can care for them. On the front burner, you'll make them chicken soup and perhaps even spoon-feed it to them. Holding them in your arms, you'll comfort them. You'll pray. You'll stay up through the night. You'll go to the pharmacy to get medicine, paying whatever you have to. You'll travel far so they can see the best medical specialists. Your unyielding desire will be for them to get better. And you will continue to love them through all of this, even when they're cranky or uncooperative.

Now think about your heavenly Father. Does He love you any less? Is His desire for you to get better? What do you think He wants to do for you?

Sometimes His love seems to be absent. Suffering might prompt us to doubt His love, but it can never negate the reality of His love. Later, we'll explore many reasons God might allow a person to suffer for a season. Pain has purpose. It's sometimes necessary. You understand this when you let your child get vaccinated with a sharp needle, or when you compel them to swallow medicine that tastes terrible, or when you consent to their body being pierced by a surgeon's knife. You wouldn't hesitate to inject them with epinephrine in the event of a serious allergic reaction. You allow your child to be inflicted with such pain because of how much you love them. You know that the temporary pain will benefit them, even if it makes them kick and scream.

God loves us dearly, even when He allows suffering into our lives. God isn't some aloof deity oblivious to our pain. He sees our every tear. He hears our every moan. He feels our every ache. He senses our anguish. God only lets us suffer for as long as there is beneficial purpose in it. His ultimate plan is to permanently end our suffering when we join Him in heaven.

When Jesus walked this earth, He demonstrated His love for people by healing a great multitude of them. Whenever God heals someone today, He presently exhibits His love for humankind. God's love is so vast that He often heals those who don't even acknowledge Him. While contemplating God's love, we can appreciate His *desire* to heal us. If He doesn't quickly heal us, we must not doubt His love. We must instead wait for healing to come, trusting that He has our best interests in mind every moment.

Father God loved us so much that He sent His own Son, Jesus, to die for our sins. Jesus loved us so much, He was willing to die an excruciating death to provide a way for us to be reconciled to the Father. Neither the love of the Father nor the love of Jesus has ever been equalled by the love of anyone else in history. View your present situation through the lens of God's love—a love that is far greater than we can ever experience, receive, or bestow in the realm of human interaction.

When you pray aloud for the healing of others, pray that they will feel the love of God flowing through you. I sensed the love of God when my uncle and my pastor prayed for the healing of my crippling muscle disease. I have felt that same divine love when my husband, mother, adult children, or others have prayed for me during later health challenges. Family members have told me, with tears trickling down, how loved by God they have felt when someone prayed for them.

Kindness

The Lord is "filled with kindness" (Psalm 145:17b, NLT).

Jesus displayed the kindness of God. We can read, for example, about Jesus visiting the home of Simon, a leper, who lived in Bethany (Matthew 26:6). Other people treated lepers with fear and cruelty. Full-blown leprosy grotesquely altered its victims, often causing twisted bone structure (such as curled fingers), tumour-like growths on the skin, and collapse of the nose.[5] Lepers had to live outside the village walls because their "unclean" disease was highly contagious. Jesus put Himself at risk when He entered the home of Simon. Some disciples were with Him, and they were placed in peril, too. It took both courage and kindness to visit Simon. Because Bethany was a long walk from Jerusalem, Jesus and His disciples likely stayed for a few meals, and at least one night, prolonging their risky contact with Simon's infectious bacteria.

God's kindness also comes to visit us. We might feel it when our pain dissipates or our sickness abates. God's kindness might flow through the people He places around us in times of injury, sickness, or surgery: caring doctors and nurses, friends who send encouraging cards or texts, and family members who sit by our bedside.

God's kindness can also bless caregivers. When my husband was in the hospital, a friend came to my door on a chilly winter night, hand-delivering freshly baked bread and a container of hot, homemade soup. I literally *tasted* God's kindness that evening.

Compassion

God has enormous compassion for the sick and the suffering. In Old Testament days, God empowered Elijah to raise the dead son of a widow back to life (1 Kings 17:17–24). On another occasion, God used Elisha to heal the leprosy of a Syrian general named Naaman (2 Kings 5:14).

And then came Jesus. He compassionately healed countless people. Matthew 9:35–36 tells us that Jesus travelled to many places, "… healing every disease and every affliction. When he saw the crowds, he had compassion for them…"

Matthew 14:14 describes one such occasion: "When he [Jesus] went ashore [at the Sea of Galilee] he saw a great crowd, and he had compassion on them and healed their sick." On another occasion, Jesus, filled with compassion, healed a leper (Mark 1:42).

Jesus was so compassionate that He dared to heal a man's shrivelled hand on the Sabbath day, knowing that the religious leaders would harshly criticize Him for breaking the Jewish Sabbath law (Luke 6:6–8).

When the religious leaders later sent men to unjustly arrest Jesus, one of His disciples struck the High Priest's servant with a sword, cutting off his ear. With compassion, Jesus "touched his ear and healed him" (Luke 22:51c).

The Lord wants to be compassionate toward us too.

Empathy

No strangers to pain, both Father God and Jesus empathize with our suffering.

When Jesus heard that His good friend Lazarus had died, He wept. The life of Jesus was sin-free, but not pain-free.

Jesus suffered immensely in the final hours of His life. Imagine how He must have felt when He was brutally whipped, forced to wear a crown of sharp thorns, and ordered to carry a heavy wooden cross. Imagine Him being hung on that rough cross, with giant nails penetrating His hands and feet, left there for hours in the heat of the day, with only bitter sips of sour vinegar to drink. I believe that Father God also suffered horribly as He watched those events unfold, knowing that He had chosen that painful path for His Son. They both endured that suffering for our sakes.

Pause to reflect on how much empathy Father God and Jesus His Son must feel right now for your pain and suffering. The tender heart of God aches for us.

Mercy

God has revealed that He can be merciful. David wrote: "Surely [His] goodness and mercy shall follow me all the days of my life..." (Psalm 23:6a). Are you willing to believe, like David, that *surely* the Lord wants to grant you His mercy throughout your whole life?

In Psalm 30, we learn that David had been deathly ill. He prayed for God's mercy, and God healed him:

O Lord my God, I cried to you for help, and you restored my
health. You brought me up from the grave, O Lord... You kept me

from falling into the pit of death… I cried out to you, O Lord. I
begged the Lord for mercy, saying, "What will you gain if I die, if
I sink into the grave? Can my dust praise you? Can it tell of your
faithfulness? Hear me, Lord, and have mercy on me. Help me, O
Lord." You have turned my mourning into joyful dancing. You
have taken away my clothes of mourning and clothed me with joy,
that I might sing praises to you and not be silent. O Lord my God,
I will give you thanks forever!

Psalm 30:2–3, 8–12, NLT

David later wrote this song of praise: "The Lord is gracious and merciful, slow to anger and abounding in steadfast love. The Lord is good to all, and his mercy is over all that he has made" (Psalm 145:8–9).

The mercy of God shone brightly in the character and actions of His Son, Jesus, when He lived on earth. Sick people often appealed to the mercy of Jesus. Mark 10:46–52 tells the story of a blind man named Bartimaeus. One day, after Jesus and His followers left Jericho, they came near Bartimaeus, who was sitting by the roadside begging. Someone in the crowd told the blind man that Jesus was passing alongside him. The beggar called out: "… Jesus, Son of David, have mercy on me!" (v. 47b).

How did Jesus respond? Was He irritated by the blind beggar's plea? Was He so tired of the crowd pressing around Him that He had no energy left for the beggar? Was He in too much of a rush to react? No. Jesus, stopping in front of Bartimaeus, gave him His undivided attention. Jesus asked the blind man a generously open-ended question: "What do you want me to do for you?" (v. 51a). Bartimaeus answered that he wanted to recover his sight. With mercy, Jesus healed the blind man right on the spot.

Jesus is still asking suffering people who seek His mercy: What do you want Me to do for you? Do you ever hear Him asking *you* that? What is your answer going to be? What do you want Him to do for you? Are you willing to tell Him your need? Believe He *is* speaking to you, here and now. Can you detect His mercy? Do you think He has less mercy to extend to you than the mercy He offered the blind beggar?

Here's a similar example of the mercy of Jesus:

> *Two blind men were sitting by the roadside, and when they heard that Jesus was going by, they shouted, "Lord, Son of David, have mercy on us!" ... Jesus stopped and called them. "What do you want me to do for you?" he asked. "Lord," they answered, "we want our sight." Jesus had compassion on them and touched their eyes. Immediately they received their sight and followed him.*
>
> Matthew 20:30–34, NIV

I suspect that Jesus must have had a reputation for being merciful by this point. Perhaps stories about His earlier healings had gone viral (the old-fashioned way). Maybe the two blind men had even heard about the healing of Bartimaeus.

God has mercy on us even though none of us deserves it. We have all sinned and fallen short of what He requires, yet He cares about our afflictions.

The apostle Paul instructed Christians to seek God's mercy: "Let us then with confidence draw near to the throne of grace, that we may receive mercy and find grace to help in time of need" (Hebrews 4:16).

God is especially merciful to those who are merciful. Jesus taught: "Blessed are the merciful, for they shall receive mercy" (Matthew 5:7).

We can notice expressions of His mercy even before He heals us. When we're in the hospital, some medical personnel might turn out to be supportive fellow believers. God's mercy might show up when our hospital room has a good view. Perhaps our room is blessedly private, or we get to share a room with a person who provides good company.

By His mercy, God can speed up medical care. I noted God's mercy when I brought my husband to the emergency wing of our local hospital (after he told me he was experiencing the worst headache of his life). Remarkably, there was only *one* person ahead of us in line (quite a miracle in a busy urban hospital, where the wait to be seen by an emergency doctor can take hours). The same thing happened to me when I had to go to emergency on one occasion.

We can't expect to encounter *all* these mercies every time we find ourselves in a hospital, but let's be thankful for every single mercy, however small, which comes our way while we wait for His healing mercy.

I love this passage: "The steadfast love of the Lord never ceases; his mercies never come to an end; they are new every morning; great is your [the Lord's] faithfulness" (Lamentations 3:22–23). How comforting that we can expect fresh mercy from God every day. I wonder how He will extend His mercy to me and to you this day?

Sometimes when I pray for others, asking God for mercy, I confess that I don't know what His mercy will look like. If I'm praying for a person who is suffering to a significant degree, I recognize that God's greatest mercy might be to take that person from this life of pain to their eternal life with Him. God's concept of mercy is sometimes greater than our ability to comprehend it. At times, I simply pray, "Father, pour out your great mercy, whatever that looks like in this situation." Our hearts ache and break when a loved one is sick or suffering. We can cry out for His mercy and it *will* come to everyone involved, but let's not presuppose what that mercy will look like.

Agnes Sanford, famous for her healing ministry, wrote about the final years of her husband. When he became sick, she prayed for him, and he lived for another three-and-a-half years. After her husband suffered a major stroke, Agnes stopped praying for his healing. She wondered if further prolonging his life might also prolong his suffering. She trusted that God was in a better position to decide what was best for her husband.[6] We must all be ready to hand our loved ones over to our merciful God. We wish our loved ones would live forever, but we don't want them to live in constant pain. (If they are believers, they *will* live forever, just not on this earth, and no longer in pain.)

Surely His mercy will follow us all of the days of our lives, here and beyond.

Grace

Psalm 145:13c reveals that God "is gracious in all he does" (NLT). Grace can be described as God's unmerited favour toward us.

Let's never take that grace for granted. Let's never abuse it. We shouldn't lightly seek God's grace while cherishing sin. God's grace flows down to us because of the death of His Son on the cross. That grace cost much. We must be in awe of such grace and always treat it with due reverence and respect. While God doesn't expect us to be perfect (we *will* fail Him over and over), He *does* expect us to repent of any sin and to renew our resolve to obey Him. Let's have honourable and honouring hearts when we come to Him to receive His grace (Hebrews 4:16).

Let's remember to acknowledge God's grace in the matter of healing. It's tempting to sometimes think we have good health because of all that *we* do in our own strength, such as exercising, eating nutritiously, or seeking out the best medical care. Those actions benefit our health, but ultimately, both health and healing are gifts that come to us by the grace of God. We can develop pride in the state of our health as much as we can develop pride regarding our finances, possessions, careers, intelligence, or beauty. May we never forget: we experience health and healing because God chooses to deal graciously with us.

Remembering God's Character

I encourage you to remain mindful of God's character as you go through your healing journey. Embrace a healing theology that is consistent with God's revealed character. As you deepen your belief that God has the wonderful character qualities we have mentioned, you'll also grow in your belief that God cares about you and wants to heal you.

Ask Him for healing on the basis of His love, kindness, compassion, empathy, mercy, and grace. Feel the warmth and comfort of His presence while you wait for healing to come. God loves you. He feels your pain. He wants to exercise kindness and compassion. He wants to extend mercy and grace.

4

GOD AS GIVER

Our loving God gives us many gifts. He's the greatest giver ever. Here are just some of God's most amazing gifts: life on this earth; salvation; health and healing; and eternal life with Him, for those who accept the gift of salvation. In this chapter, I want to highlight the gifts of life and eternal life.

The Time-Limited Gift of Life

Life is a gift we can make the most of and enjoy. We must, however, address the reality that God's gift of life has a limit. Each life has an expiry date. The gift of life that you have received isn't identical to the life that I have received. The issue of how long we each get to live on this earth has to be considered alongside our study of God's healing power. We must accept the fact that God will heal us up to a certain point in time, and then death will come.

We learn from Psalm 139:16 that, even while we were being formed in the womb, God knew about every day we'd spend on earth. He wrote down, in His book, the tally of our days. God knew the end from the beginning. He knows how our life will unfold, including the decisions we'll make along the way that will affect our lifespan. Before the date of our birth, He already knew the exact date of our death. Ecclesiastes 3:1 teaches that there is a time to be born and a time to die. Job rightly stated: "You [God] have decided the length of our lives. You know how many months we will live, and we are not given a minute longer" (Job 14:5, NLT).

Jesus, now seated with the Father in heaven, holds the keys to death (Revelation 1:18). He unlocks the door of death in His sovereign timing.

Some Bible verses talk about living a long life or a full life. Abraham, for example, "died at a ripe old age, having lived a long and satisfying life" (Genesis 25:8a, NLT). One psalmist scribed: "Because he holds fast to me [the Lord] in love, I will deliver him; I will protect him because he knows my name... With long life I [the Lord] will satisfy him and show him my salvation" (Psalm 91:14, 16). Jesus taught: "The thief [our enemy] comes only to steal and kill and destroy. I [Jesus] have come that they might have life, and have it to the full" (John 10:10, NIV).

Other verses make specific reference to length of life. Adam and the generations just after him lived hundreds of years. Noah died at 950 years old (Genesis 9:29). Age spans began to shorten after Noah. Abraham lived to the age of 175 (Genesis 25:7). His wife, Sarah, reached 127 (Genesis 23:1). Joseph died at 110 years old (Genesis 50:22).

Moses wrote this declaration of the Lord in Genesis 6:3: "My Spirit will not put up with humans for such a long time [as He had in the past], for they are only mortal flesh. In the future, their normal lifespan will be no more than 120 years" (NLT). Moses lived to be 120 years, with eyes "undimmed" and "vigor unabated" (Deuteronomy 34:7). I could find no record of any biblical figure born after Moses living beyond 120. The upper age limit to *this* day remains about 120 years, despite all the advances in medical science. The *Guinness Book of World Records* doesn't acknowledge anyone living beyond 120 except for one French woman who died in 1997 at the supposed age of 122. As 2019 begins, not one person alive *today*, out of the more than seven billion people on earth, can establish that they are older than 115.[7] I find it amazing that God set an upper limit for lifespan many thousands of years ago, as recorded by Moses in the book of Genesis, which remains in place to this day.

One final biblical reference to expected lifespan can be found in Psalm 90:10a: "The years of our life are seventy, or even by reason of strength eighty." Over time, genes mutated, pollution arose, pathogens developed, and disease spread, impairing health and preventing most people from reaching the upper lifespan of 120.

It's tempting to extract that single verse, Psalm 90:10, out of the Bible and to assume it applies to everyone. I'm now in my sixties. I pray that I live at least ten or twenty more years. I'm not certain, however, that Psalm 90:10 creates a specific promise. Perhaps it's more of a general statement as to how long most people will likely live.

It's reasonable to say in modern Western society that most people will live until they're seventy or eighty, but some will die before then, and some will live longer.

We're not *entitled* to seventy or eighty years. We're not *guaranteed* to live that long. The person who believes such entitlement exists will be greatly confused whenever someone they know dies younger than seventy. Perhaps their faith in God will be rocked.

I conducted an interesting informal survey on the lifespans of some famous Christians from different theological backgrounds, nations, occupations, and periods of history. I quite randomly picked the names of two dozen well-known Christians as they came to mind. They died at the following ages from failing health (not from war, martyrdom, or any other non-health-related cause):

4th century	Caesar Constantine (ruler of the Roman Empire)	65
5th century	St. Augustine (author of theological books)	76
14th century	John Wycliffe (translator of the Latin Bible into English)	53
15th century	Johannes Gutenberg (printing press inventor/Bible printer)	70

16th century	Martin Luther (father of the Protestant Reformation)	63
17th century	Galileo (pioneer of modern physics)	78
18th century	Sir Isaac Newton (physicist and mathematician)	84
18th century	John Wesley (well-known British preacher)	88
18th century	Charles Wesley (John's brother, also a preacher)	81
18th century	George Frideric Handel (composer of musical masterpieces)	74
18th century	Isaac Watts (composer of over six hundred English hymns)	74
19th century	John Newton (ex-slave trader who wrote "Amazing Grace")	83
19th century	William Wilberforce (he fought to abolish the slave trade)	73
19th century	William Carey ("father" of modern missions)	73
19th century	Catherine Booth (co-founder of the Salvation Army)	61
19th century	Charles Spurgeon (well-known British preacher)	57
20th century	Billy Sunday (pro baseball player turned preacher)	83
20th century	Amy Carmichael (missionary in India)	84
20th century	C. S. Lewis (author of many Christian classics)	64
20th century	A. W. Tozer (author and pastor)	66

20th century	Oswald J. Smith (well-known Canadian pastor)	96
20th century	Mother Teresa (served the poor in India)	87
21st century	Ruth Bell Graham (wife of Billy Graham)	87
21st century	Billy Graham (world-famous evangelist)	99

Twenty-two of those twenty-four men and women lived past age sixty; seventeen (more than two-thirds) lived past seventy; and ten (more than one-third) lived past eighty or ninety. The longevity of many of them surprises me, since sixteen of them (two-thirds) lived before the year 1900, and some were missionaries in disease-ravaged countries. Their lifespans differ by decades, demonstrating that none of us are guaranteed to live until some magic age. The average age of death of those twenty-four people is 75.6 years. This average fits within the general observation, contained in Psalm 90:10, written thousands of years ago, that God's people would live until age seventy or eighty.

I believe that we will live the *full* life that we have been ordained to live, however long that is, *if* we choose obedience to God. Moses told God's people:

> … *Take to heart all the words by which I am warning you today, that you may command them to your children, that they may be careful to do all the words of this law. For it is no empty word for you, but your very life, and by this word you shall live long…*
> Deuteronomy 32:46–47

Similarly, Proverbs 3:1–2 promises: "… let your heart keep my commandments, for length of days and years of life and peace they will add to you." Proverbs 3:16 states: "Long life is in her [godly wisdom's] right hand…"

Only God knows what a full and long life will mean for you and for me.

I suspect that a full life involves living out the fullness of God's plans and purposes. He has different plans and purposes for each one of us, and they will take varying amounts of time. I don't believe He'll take us from this earth until we've finished the tasks set for us.

I'm talking about God-ordained tasks, not our bucket lists. If we're spending our waning years *only* focusing on ticking things off *our* list (visiting Mongolia for no particular reason, trying skydiving, or learning to speak Swahili for the fun of it), God may have no reason to keep us here. If, however, we're busy with God's purposes, God will likely sustain us until the plans He has appointed are fulfilled.

To reach our full lifespan, we must take reasonably good care of our health, to the best of our ability. God might unlock the door of death sooner than He planned *if* we're foolish and do things that compromise our health. We can *shorten* the fullness of our days. An extreme example of this would be suicide. Eating poorly hastens the timing of our departure from this life. God already knew about such destructive choices when He recorded the number of our days long before our birth.

Right spiritual choices help us to live out the fullness of our days. I'm delighted every time I read about a study that shows that praying, church-attending Christians generally live longer than those who don't develop those habits.[8] God also foreknew those good choices when He recorded the number of our days long ago.

Can we do anything to *extend* our lifespan? An intriguing story is told in 2 Kings 20:1–6. That story begins with King Hezekiah being very ill and near death. The prophet Isaiah came to him with these ominous words: "Thus says the Lord, 'Set your house in order, for you shall die; you shall not recover'" (v. 1b). The king turned his face to the wall and privately pleaded with God: "Now, O Lord, please remember how I have walked before you in faithfulness and with a whole heart, and have done what is good in your sight" (v. 3a). After King Hezekiah finished praying, he wept bitterly. Perhaps he felt his terminal illness was unfair.

The prophet Isaiah was leaving the palace when God spoke further to him:

Turn back, and say to Hezekiah the leader of my people, Thus says the Lord, the God of David your father: I have heard your prayer; I have seen your tears. Behold, I will heal you. On the third day you shall go up to the house of the Lord, and I will add fifteen years to your life. (vv. 5–6a)

All of that came to pass. God had known all along, even before Hezekiah was born, what Hezekiah would petition and that He would grant that petition. I believe that the number of days allotted to Hezekiah at the time he was conceived would have taken into account God's foreknowledge of the events we have just described.

King Hezekiah's plea was based on the life he'd led. Pause to consider 2 Kings 20:3a again: "Now, O Lord, please remember how I have walked before you in faithfulness and with a whole heart, and have done what is good in your sight." I imagine that this is the best argument any of us can make to live longer on this earth.

It seems that God still listens to some prayerful petitions for the extension of life (having known from the beginning of time that such petitions would be made and granted), although not everyone will get fifteen more years like Hezekiah.

Former U.S. Secretary of State Condoleezza Rice, who served under President George W. Bush, recounts an interesting story. Condoleezza was fifteen years old when her mother received a breast cancer diagnosis. An only child, Condoleezza had been close to her mother. The thought of losing her mother, while still a teenager, must have been devastating. Condoleezza and her father prayed together, asking that God would grant her mother an extra fifteen years of life. They pleaded for Mrs. Rice to see Condoleezza grow into adulthood. God mercifully answered that prayer. Mrs. Rice died when Condoleezza was thirty years old, exactly fifteen years later.[9]

I have a similar story to tell from my own family. In 1999, my father suffered two massive heart attacks a few hours apart. The attacks left him in critical condition. At the hospital, he underwent testing that determined that two left arteries were substantially blocked. One was 100 percent blocked; the other was 80 percent obstructed. The back-to-back heart attacks had caused significant damage to some heart muscles. The cardiac team decided that there was no point in performing stent procedures or open-heart surgery on the compromised arteries, because the surrounding muscles were too weak to pump blood through those arteries. The doctors couldn't do much to improve my dad's diseased and damaged heart. They could only stabilize him.

My whole family prayed for my dad. My mom was with my dad during both heart attacks, so she'd prayed for him, from the outset, that he would live and not die. She remembers quoting Bible verses as she stood by my dad in the emergency treatment room, surrounded by doctors and nurses. One of the doctors wanted my mom to leave the room; another said she could stay.

My sister later encouraged our family to pray that our dad would live a further fifteen years. Considering that our dad had been a fairly heavy smoker for fifty-five years, and that he was almost seventy years old, her prayer suggestion struck me as audacious. A further fifteen years seemed highly improbable from a medical point of view. The cardiac team hadn't expected my dad to live through the first *night* after his dual heart attacks, never mind fifteen more years. One cardiologist declared that it was a miracle that my dad lived at all after his dual attacks, considering the extent of the heart damage.

I now write this twenty years later. I report with gratitude that God graciously brought my dad through that life-threatening medical crisis. Since then, God has also brought him through a week in ICU for a serious gastric bleed and through two years of chemotherapy treatment for lymphoma, a cancer of the bone marrow.

Up to the age of eighty-six, my father worked part time. Until recently, my parents travelled far and wide, taking weeks-long cruises. Not long ago, my parents downsized their home, but they still live independently. On many levels, and for several years, my dad's health after his cardiac crisis was better than it had been before. His decision to stop smoking, and other positive lifestyle adjustments, certainly helped. God healed my father to the point where he could go on living a long and full life.

God has extended the lives of others, too, beyond what their doctors expected. Years ago, an older friend named Bev received a diagnosis of breast cancer, which had metastasized to other parts of her body, including her brain. Bev started attending a Bible study hosted in my home on the topic of healing.

As I got to know Bev, I grew in my admiration of her walk with God. She had a strong belief in His Word. She chose to trust God, no matter what her medical reports said. She prayed ardently. She humbly requested prayer from others and remained involved at church. She cared about others. She ministered to me.

She lived about a dozen years with stage-four cancer, including many years after her last medical treatment, with reasonable quality of life and remarkable energy—far surpassing the amount of time her oncologist had prognosed. God sustained her for a long season and used her to bless and encourage many others. I'll never forget her exceptional desire to follow her Lord, and His gift to her of extended life and fruitfulness.

Although we have some part to play in our length of days, God remains sovereign over the date of our birth and the date of our death. Only He knows when we have fulfilled the roles and the tasks He's created for us.

Our bodies are programmed for both life *and* death. God set those opposing dynamics in motion from the moment of conception. While our bodies are programmed to grow, function, and heal themselves from many kinds of dysfunction, they are also programmed to age and move relentlessly toward death. Our health, strength, and energy will vary over the years, but there will be eventual decline.

Our bodies are like the GPS system in a car. As soon as we input a destination into the GPS, the system is programmed to end at that point. Until the end is reached, however, the system will be full of "life." GPS directions will tell us to turn left, or right, or move forward. When the end point is reached, the GPS instructions will cease, and the driver will bring the vehicle to a stop. The system can handle being preprogrammed for a period of *activity* and then for the *stop* of all activity. In a similar way, God has programmed us, from our very beginning, for both life and death. We can enjoy life for a period of time while we're moving certainly toward death.

King Solomon wrote: "None of us can hold back our spirit from departing. None of us has the power to prevent the day of our death" (Ecclesiastes 8:8a, NLT).

Perhaps some of our loved ones left this earth earlier than we would have liked. Is it possible that God spared them from something yet to come? Isaiah 57:1–2 states: "The righteous man perishes… devout men are taken away, while no one understands. For the righteous man is taken away from calamity; he enters into peace…"

God has His reasons, which we may or may not understand, for ordaining a particular end point for each one of our mortal lives.

James 4:14–15 tells us:

> *… you do not know what tomorrow will bring. What is your life?*
> *For you are a mist that appears for a little time and then vanish-*
> *es… you ought to say, "If the Lord wills, we will live*
> *and do this or that."*

At some point, our bodies will shut down and God will not interfere. Some people may seem to die peacefully in their sleep, but in reality, they have gone through a cardiac arrest, or a brain seizure, or some other malfunction that has ended their life.

In 2 Kings 13:14, we read: "… Elisha had fallen sick with the illness of which he was to die…" Like the great prophet Elisha, we may also have a sickness unto death one day. God may heal us over and over, but one day He will choose not to heal us.

Evangelist Oral Roberts survived a few heart attacks, but later died at age ninety-one of pneumonia,[10] his sickness unto death. He lived a full and long life, experienced God's healing power on many occasions, and served as a channel of it for others. In the end, God didn't heal his final sickness.

Let's continue to pray for healing as long as we and our loved ones are alive, while recognizing that we cannot control the timing or manner of anyone's death.

The Gift of Eternal Life

Death is not really the terminal point. Death may end the *earthly* sojourn of believers, but it does not end *us*. An endless life awaits us.

Consider these wonderful words of the apostle Paul:

> *When the perishable put on the imperishable, and the mortal puts on immortality, then shall come to pass the saying that is written: "Death is swallowed up in victory." "O death, where is your victory? O death, Where is your sting?"… But thanks be to God, who gives us the victory through our Lord Jesus Christ.*
>
> 1 Corinthians 15:54–55, 57

Paul also wrote:

> *For to me to live is Christ, and to die is gain. If I am to live in the flesh, that means fruitful labor for me. Yet which I shall choose I cannot tell. I am hard pressed between the two. My desire is to depart and be with Christ, for that is far better.*
>
> Philippians 1:21–23

Death is the portal into our eternal lives, which will be far better.

Maybe an unsaved loved one has died and you're disturbed about their destiny. Perhaps, without you knowing about it, they made their peace with God in the final days, hours, or even minutes of their life.

Don't let that uncertainty rob you of your present peace or distract you from appreciating the gift of eternal life you have accepted. Or maybe you suffered the loss of a young child. I encourage you to read the story of King David and the loss of his infant, recorded in 2 Samuel 12:15–23, which suggests children too young to make a spiritual choice will go to heaven and await us there.

If God wants to give us such magnificent gifts as life and eternal life, is it too hard to believe that He wants to give us good health and healing in this life? Although He may allow seasons of suffering, and although our health will not likely be perfect, dare we believe that He wants us to have reasonable quality of life most of our years? Dare we ask the generous giver of life and eternal life to give us a good measure of health and healing until we reach the fullness of our days? As we ask, let us remember that health is a *gift* (not a right) graciously given by the giver of all good things.

5

GOD'S INTENTION

I love the Latin expression *Deo Volente*. It can be translated: as God wishes; as God wills; as God intends; or as God resolves. I don't know what God's will might be regarding many matters, but can we know His will regarding *some* matters? Has He spoken enough in His Word about particular topics that we can know what He has generally willed in *those* areas of life?

I believe God has expressed His will very clearly in some areas. God doesn't want anyone to lie or steal or commit adultery.

Has He expressed His will regarding the healing of the sick and the suffering?

One afternoon, a series of visitors came through a teenage patient's hospital room, where I was present. The first visitor stood beside me and prayed boldly for the patient, plainly asking God to heal him. The next few, who happened to stand on the other side of the bed, prayed for God to heal him *if* it was His will. The young teen expressed his confusion after all the visitors had left. Why those duelling prayers? Did God want to heal him or not?

What is God's will in this matter of healing? I believe, very simply, that it is God's general will to heal all who ask for healing. We can, however, create obstacles to the fulfilment of God's will by being disobedient, holding certain theological mindsets, becoming impatient, giving up, or neglecting to pray. We'll talk more about these and other obstacles to healing.

If we're not obstructing our own healing, I believe that God wants to heal us, at least to some degree. Even doctors do their best to facilitate the healing of every patient who comes to them. No doctor has ever said to me, "I don't want to help you heal." Surely God cares about us more than human doctors.

Here's a key passage that supports God's willingness to heal:

> *When he [Jesus] came down from the mountain, great crowds followed him. And behold, a leper came to him and knelt before him, saying, "Lord, if you will, you can make me clean." And Jesus stretched out his hand and touched him, saying, "I will; be clean." And immediately his leprosy was cleansed.*
>
> Matthew 8:1–3

Jesus was willing to heal that man. He *said* so and then He did so. Mark 1:40–42 records a similar story:

> *A man with leprosy came to him [Jesus] and begged him on his knees, "If you are willing, you can make me clean…" He [Jesus] reached out his hand and touched the man. "I am willing," he said. "Be clean!" Immediately the leprosy left him and he was cleansed.* (NIV)

Do you think He is any less willing to heal you? On what basis do you believe that? Can you dare to ask Him now, "Lord, are You willing to heal *me*?" Listen for His answer as you continue to read.

"I am willing," Jesus said in both of these gospel accounts. Can you find any story in scripture in which Jesus expressly said "I am *not* willing" to a person seeking healing? I have looked with diligence and cannot find such a story.

Why, then, should we ask Jesus *if* He is willing to heal us when He has already declared that He *is* willing? It seems that many people attach more weight to the leper's mindset (*if* you will) than to the unequivocal mindset of Jesus (I *will*).

Jesus didn't always verbally express His willingness to heal, but He actively demonstrated such willingness over and over again. Jesus often healed all who came to Him for healing on a particular day in a particular place, even when a large crowd bombarded Him (see, for example, Matthew 4:23–24; 9:35; 12:15–16; 14:14). Jesus expressed His willingness to heal with His actions far more than with His words.

At one point, Jesus told His followers that He had come to earth to perform the will of the Father (John 6:38). When Jesus healed so many people on so many occasions, surely such healing manifested the will of the Father.

Maybe you're not convinced. Is there some middle ground between the "*if* it is God's will to heal" position of some and the "I believe it *is* God's will to heal" position that I take? Perhaps you can be comfortable with this proposed middle ground: Instead of praying for healing *if* it is God's will, you can consider praying for healing *in accordance with* God's will. The phrase "if it is God's will" lacks conviction. It doesn't contain a declaration of faith or desire. It doesn't give rise to a defined prayer request. The second suggested phrase, "in accordance with God's will," doesn't sound so tentative or vague.

Those who prefer the word "if" in their prayer might argue that they don't want to impinge on God's sovereignty by assuming what His will is. But we don't violate God's sovereignty when asking for healing "in accordance with His will." The latter wording fully submits to God's sovereignty.

Your Kingdom Come, Your Will Be Done

We can also pray using the words of the Lord's Prayer, given to us by Jesus: "… Our Father in heaven, hallowed be your name. Your kingdom come, your will be done, on earth as it is in heaven" (Matthew 6:9–10).

That last sentence can be paraphrased: Your will be done here on earth in accordance with what You have planned and purposed in heaven.

The phrase "your will be done" follows "your kingdom come." What does God's kingdom look like when it comes down to us? While walking among humankind, Jesus said that the kingdom of God was "near" or "at hand." We find this phrase several times in the gospel accounts. As He began His healing ministry, Jesus declared: "… The time is fulfilled, and the kingdom of God is at hand…" (Mark 1:15). The many healings He performed thereafter gave the watching crowds a glimpse into God's glorious kingdom.

In Matthew 10:7–8a, Jesus instructed His twelve disciples: "… proclaim as you go, saying, 'The kingdom of heaven is at hand.' Heal the sick…" Healing of the sick demonstrated God's kingdom being at hand.

In Luke 10:9, Jesus told seventy-two of His followers to travel in pairs from town to town. Each time they entered a new town, Jesus wanted them to "heal the sick in it and say to them, 'The kingdom of God has come near to you.'"

Notice that Jesus *didn't* say: "Heal them after you first find out if it is My will to heal them. Find out who is sick in each village and come back and discuss them with Me, and I will tell you whom to heal." No, Jesus said to go and heal the sick to reveal one aspect of what God's kingdom looks like.

Throughout the gospels, healing was visible evidence of the presence of God's kingdom come down to earth. I encourage you to remember the verses describing God's kingdom on earth (and all of the healing that occurred) the next time you pray in accordance with the Lord's Prayer, "Your kingdom come, your will be done, on earth as it is in heaven."

In this present world (where many resist God's kingdom), we know that His kingdom has not been fully ushered in. We can get only a taste of it, just as people did in the time of Jesus. Many billions don't welcome God's kingdom. But *we* can be among those who still pray for His kingdom to come here and His will to be done. We can watch for the sick to be healed as one visible manifestation of His kingdom come down.

Paul's Thorn

Some argue that Paul's "thorn in the flesh" proves that God isn't always willing to heal. Paul prayed for it to be removed, but it still bothered him, when he wrote:

> *... to keep me from becoming conceited, I was given a thorn in my flesh, a messenger of Satan, to torment me. Three times I pleaded with the Lord to take it away from me. But he said to me, "My grace is sufficient for you, for my power is made perfect in weakness." Therefore I will boast all the more gladly about my weaknesses, so that Christ's power may rest on me. That is why, for Christ's sake, I delight in weaknesses, in insults, in hardships, in persecutions, in difficulties. For when I am weak, then I am strong.*
>
> 2 Corinthians 12:7b–10, NIV

I don't believe that Paul's "thorn in the flesh" was a physical thorn (i.e., something like a thorn from a rose stem). Doctors existed in those days. Removing a thorn would not have been a difficult task. Luke, a friend and travelling companion of Paul, was a physician (Colossians 4:14) who could have treated Paul.

In the Old Testament, descriptions of thorns in the bodies of God's people referred metaphorically to their human enemies. For example, God told the Israelites to drive the Canaanites out of their land because they worshipped idols. God warned: "But if you do not drive out the inhabitants of the land, those you allow to remain will become barbs in your eyes and *thorns in your sides*. They will give you trouble..." (Numbers 33:55, NIV).

On another occasion, God warned the Israelites:

But if you turn away and ally yourselves with the survivors of
these nations that remain among you and if you intermarry with
them and associate with them, then you may be sure that the Lord
your God will no longer drive out these nations before you. Instead,
they will become snares and traps for you, whips on your backs and
thorns in your eyes, until you perish from this good land…

Joshua 23:12–13, NIV

Paul was a learned Jewish scholar before he became a Christian. He would have been well aware of the thorn references in such Old Testament passages. We can reasonably believe that Paul, in his letter to the Corinthians, was referring to his own thorn metaphorically (i.e., representing an enemy of his).

Paul described his "thorn in the flesh" as "a messenger of Satan" who tormented him. The word "messenger" sounds like a reference to a *person*, perhaps a persecutor or critic. Paul concluded that God allowed this "messenger" to stick around to keep Paul from becoming proud. A messenger delivers words. We don't know what words this tormenting messenger spoke, but they weakened Paul, who turned to God for strength.

It seems strange to me to think of a physical thorn from a prickly plant as a "messenger." I find it equally strange to characterize a sickness or disease as a "messenger." It makes more sense to interpret the "messenger of Satan" as meaning a persecutor. To buttress this interpretation, I note that verse ten (three verses later) refers to persecution.

The Bible usually refers to sickness and disease expressly. There is no reason that Paul wouldn't explicitly refer to sickness, if sickness were his problem, instead of using words like "thorn in the flesh" or "messenger of Satan."

Paul had faith that God wanted to heal people. When on the island of Malta, for example, he prayed for the chief official's father to be healed. That man's fever and dysentery then left him. Other sick people in Malta came to Paul and were also healed (Acts 28:8–9). If Paul suffered from a physical ailment that God hadn't healed, how could he have had enough faith to successfully pray for the healing of the sick in Malta?

For all those reasons, I believe that Paul's phrase "thorn in the flesh" was a metaphor, akin to similar metaphors in Old Testament passages, denoting a problematic person who was a distraction and a danger. I do not think that Paul's thorn was an illness, condition, or injury that God refused to heal.

I know and respect mature Christians who believe that Paul's thorn *was* a physical problem. Some Bible commentators take the same position. Paul's letter to the Galatians mentioned a "bodily ailment" (Galatians 4:13), which might or might not have been the same thing as the thorn. Maybe it was a separate matter. Either way, neither the thorn nor the ailment stopped Paul's tremendously effective lifelong ministry.

Perhaps Paul kept praying. Perhaps he was eventually healed (or delivered) of whatever ailed him. No one can say for sure whether Paul suffered for a season of time, or permanently, from the "thorn" and "ailment."

Whatever the nature and duration of Paul's thorn or ailment, don't let either convince you that God isn't willing to heal you. Hundreds of verses describe God healing people. I suspect He eventually healed and delivered Paul too.

God's Covenant with His People

In the Old Testament, God made many covenants with His people. A covenant is a formal expression of intention. Some covenants were so significant that God gave Himself a new name (evoking a particular identity revealed in the covenant).

The Lord God gave Himself the name Jehovah Rapha. In Hebrew, the word "rapha" means "healer." That name appears in Exodus 15:26, where God declares: "… I am the Lord, your healer."

God uses the words "I am." God did not say He was, or might sometimes be, or will be for a limited time. He said, "I am," making

Him forever Jehovah Rapha, *in the present tense*, revealing a significant dimension of His unchanging essence and being.

Let's now look at the full covenant in Exodus 15:26:

> *... If you will diligently listen to the voice of the Lord your God,*
> *and do that which is right in his eyes, and give ear to his com-*
> *mandments and keep all his statutes, I will put none of the diseases*
> *on you that I put on the Egyptians, for I am the Lord, your healer.*

The two-sided healing covenant between God and His people can be simply summarized: If His people obeyed Him, He would provide health and healing.

As a lawyer, I'm familiar with covenants. A covenant creates a contract between two or more parties. Every party to the covenant/contract makes certain promises and undertakes certain obligations. A covenant can get derailed if one party breaches it by wilfully ignoring their part of the bargain. In Exodus 15:26, healing was offered as a *conditional* promise. The promise of healing was *contingent* on God's people fulfilling their part of the covenant (obeying God).

All of the covenants God made with His people in the time of Moses were conditional. Deuteronomy 7:9 states: "Know therefore that the Lord your God is God, the *faithful* God who *keeps covenant* and steadfast love *with those who love him* and *keep his commandments*, to a thousand generations..." This verse illustrates the two-sided nature of the various covenants God made with His people. (I invite you to notice that one thousand generations have not been born since those words were written.)

The following prayer of King Solomon also referred to both sides of the covenantal relationship: "... O Lord, God of Israel, there is no God like you, in heaven above or on earth beneath, keeping covenant and showing steadfast love to your servants who walk before you with all their heart..." (1 Kings 8:23).

Lawyers have an expression: A contract is only as good as the handshake behind it. The soundness and security of a contract depend on the honour, integrity, and trustworthiness of *both* parties shaking hands on a particular deal. I think we can all agree that God has honour, integrity, and trustworthiness. He will always uphold His end of whatever bargain He makes. Here's the significant issue: Do His people always uphold *their* end?

At the time this covenant was made, God's people were the Israelites. The New Testament now provides a new and better covenant between God and all of His people, based on what Jesus accomplished on the cross. I don't want to wade into deep theological waters regarding what changed between the old and new covenants. With respect to healing, however, I believe that the New Testament makes it clear that God still heals and He also still expects His people to obey Him.

Of course, none of us is perfect. We all stumble and fall. If we're sorry, confess our sins, and turn from them, He will be gracious to forgive them. We must try our best to obey God, but He understands our fallen nature. Thankfully, He is merciful. Because He is God, He sometimes heals even those who aren't obedient or repentant, although He has not scripturally obligated Himself to do so. Healing (or its absence) cannot be precisely equated with obedience (or its absence).

Perhaps I should reframe the question I posed as the chapter began. In my mind, the question is no longer whether God is willing to heal us. The real question is whether *we* are willing to do what is required of *us* in the healing process (and in our lives generally).

God's Sovereign Choices

I believe that God is willing to heal, but He gets to choose the *when* and the *how* and the *measure* of the healing. He gets to decide at what point suffering has fulfilled its many purposes. If you're concerned about God maintaining ultimate sovereignty over our lives, there's a lot of room for divine sovereignty in these matters. Anyone who has been seriously sick, injured, or disabled, or has gone under the surgeon's knife, has come face to face with a God they cannot control.

Sometimes healing is instant or occurs within days. Other times, it takes weeks, months, or even years. Sometimes it's gradual but continuous. Other times, it occurs in progressive stages punctuated by time periods in between. A setback might interrupt healing progress. God controls the timeline.

God also controls the method and process of healing. Our bodies have been preprogrammed by God to heal themselves to a large extent (further proof that God wants to heal us). Our bodies are equipped to drive out harmful bacteria and viruses and to fight inflammation and infection. Bones, skin, muscles, and other physical tissues have self-mending abilities. Sometimes God uses doctors, surgeries, and/ or medications to complete the healing process. On other occasions, He supernaturally intervenes in a health situation. We assist with our healing by such activities as getting rest, taking vitamins, or exercising to build up our strength again. God decides what combination of factors will result in healing in each situation.

God also decides on the measure of healing. Sometimes we're completely healed. Other times we're substantially healed, but not completely. As we age, we are often only partially healed (because natural death cannot eventually occur without some physical deterioration).

God's sovereignty also includes how long He allows each one of us to live. God won't keep healing us on this earth forever. Hebrews 9:27 informs us, quite bluntly, that it is appointed for all of us to die. If we don't die from unnatural causes, our bodies will eventually fail us.

We'll talk more about the *when*, the *how*, the *degree*, and the *duration* of healing in later chapters. One sure thing I've learned: We cannot dictate to God the timing, the method, the measure, or the longevity of our healing. We can respectfully ask for a specific outcome. We can provide our reasons and present our case, but we cannot control God's hand. He is sovereign. He is supreme. I believe that He wants to heal us, He is willing to heal us, but on His own terms.

Unless you're convinced that the time of death has come, I encourage you to believe that it is God's will to heal. Trust that He will heal, in His timing, in His way, in the measure He chooses, for as long as He chooses.

Being Confident in Our Prayers

Perhaps you wonder what all the fuss is about. Why do we need to take a position on whether or not God is generally willing to heal the sick and the suffering? Here's why: Our position will affect the nature of our prayers.

John wrote:

> *This is the confidence we have in approaching God: that if we ask anything according to his will, he hears us. And if we know that he hears us—whatever we ask—we know that we have what we asked of him.*
>
> 1 John 5:14–15, NIV

Wouldn't you like to approach God with John's level of confidence? Wouldn't you like to have that much assurance in the outcome? You can, if you either believe that it's generally God's will to heal, or if you're at least prepared to pray "in accordance with" God's will.

God's broader will is for us to work, serve, feed the hungry, help the poor, take care of one another, teach, and perform many other activities. Surely He wants us to have the strength and energy to do all of this. We may be sick and weak for a season, but I believe He wants us to have a great enough measure of health so that we can fulfill the many plans and purposes He has for us.

Andrew Murray wrote in his brilliant book, *With Christ in the School of Prayer*, that God wills many great blessings for us, but we don't receive them because *we* aren't willing to come into agreement with such blessings.[11] Do you believe that God is willing to heal you? I encourage you to settle this issue in your heart and mind.

6

God's Glory

God is glorious.
    He is *full* of glory.

He constantly *draws in* fresh glory.

God's glory *shines* when His power, character, good gifts, and good intentions are on display. Some synonyms for glory include: greatness, majesty, and eminence.

God and His works are worthy of glory. *Soli Deo Gloria.*

Jesus declared: "If you abide in me, and my words abide in you, ask whatever you wish, and it will be done for you. By this my Father is glorified..." (John 15:7–8a). When we ask for healing and it is given to us, the Father receives glory. When the crowds saw Jesus healing the blind, mute, crippled, and lame, "they glorified the God of Israel" (Matthew 15:31).

Acts 3 begins with a story about a crippled man. Peter said to him, "In the name of Jesus Christ of Nazareth, rise up and walk!" (v. 6b). As the man obeyed, he was healed. Peter advised the watching crowd that the healing occurred to bring glory to Jesus (v. 13).

God is still in the business of healing today, because healing brings Him great glory. Each healing should prompt us to glorify Him.

God wants us to exalt Him. Jesus taught us to pray: "… Our Father in heaven, hallowed be your name" (Matthew 6:9). Martin Luther and John Calvin agreed that one meaning of "hallowed" is "glorified."[12] The Lord's Prayer ends (in some ancient manuscripts) with the words: "For yours is the kingdom and the power and the glory, forever."[13] Whether or not those words were placed in the Lord's Prayer by Jesus or added by early Christians recopying manuscripts, they're certainly consistent with the rest of scripture. God's glory will last forever.

King David declared: "Ascribe to the Lord the glory due his name…" (Psalm 29:2a). When we talk about how God has healed us and healed others, we glorify Him.

Some say that suffering well and dying well bring God glory. I agree. Suffering and dying well *can* bring God glory. Not everyone suffers or dies well. Some suffer or die in anger, bitterness, self-pity, or some other state that is not Spirit-empowered.

The poet Dylan Thomas told us to rage against the dying of the light. As Christians, we should not die in rage. We should die gently and in peace when it's clear that it's our time to leave this earth. Thomas refers to the dying of the light, but for Christians, death is a journey *toward* the Light.

My maternal grandmother died (in her early nineties) in my mother's arms, with a peaceful smile on her face, with faith in God to the very end, and with hope in life eternal. She knew her destiny. She was ready to depart this world. She died well.

In Psalm 90:12, the psalmist implores God: "… teach us to number our days…" When we recognize that our days are limited, we can live well, and, when the time comes, we can die well, knowing that Jesus conquered the grave.

I have digressed. Let's resume talking about healing and how it brings God glory.

Now in exile, Brother Yun was a prominent leader in the Chinese house church network. In the 1980s and '90s, God used Yun and his wife to help catapult the once-struggling church in China to today's guesstimated one-hundred-million-strong church.

From young ages, both Yun and his wife experienced God's glorious power (to save, transform, and heal) and wanted others to experience it too. In 1974, when Yun was sixteen years old and not yet a Christian, his father developed stage-four lung cancer with metastasis in his stomach. Yun's family spent all their money seeking treatment for him, but the father's doctor told the family that the disease was terminal. He told Yun's mother to get her husband's affairs in order.

The family found themselves in a desperate situation. With no breadwinner to support them, Yun and his four starving siblings began begging other villagers for food. Yun's mother was so distraught at the prospect of being widowed (and left alone to raise five children in poverty), she even considered suicide.

At that time, no one in the family was a committed Christian. Many years before, Yun's mother had experienced a short season of Christian faith. As a young adult in the 1940s, Yun's mother had been exposed to foreign missionaries. She had loved the songs and the Bible stories they taught her.

When China came under Communist control in 1949, foreign missionaries were expelled, churches shut down, and Chinese pastors killed or imprisoned. Ordinary believers were harassed and sometimes tortured or murdered. Yun's mother struggled to maintain her nascent faith after that brutal crackdown, but without a Bible and without the fellowship of other believers, her faith eventually dissipated.

By the time her husband lay dying of advanced cancer in 1974, she had forgotten all about God. But God had not forgotten her. As she lay in bed one night, she heard a distinct voice speak to her three simple words: "Jesus loves you." She immediately got out of bed, knelt down, confessed her sins, and asked Jesus to come back into her life.

She roused her five children, including sixteen-year-old Yun, and told them what had just happened. She said that Jesus was their only hope. All of the children committed their lives to Christ right then and there. Afterward, they gathered around their father. Laying their hands on him, they prayed together for Jesus to heal their father. Over and over through that night, they prayed in united petition.

The following morning, Yun's father said that he felt better than before. He had lost his appetite months before, but that morning he wanted to eat. Over the next days, he rapidly recovered his strength. By the end of that week, his cancer was completely gone, never to return. He died a few years later of other causes.[14]

This dramatic healing so displayed God's love and power that Yun's mother and all five children continued to follow Jesus through extreme hardships. They had experienced the glory of God and would never forget it.

His father's healing particularly impacted Yun, who drew close to God in every way he could. He prayed daily. For months, he repeatedly asked God for a Bible. Two men knocked at his door one day bearing a gift of that precious book, which was a rare commodity in China at that time. Yun read his new Bible voraciously, memorizing chapter after chapter. While still a teenager, he travelled to other villages to reach them for Christ. Over the years, Yun (who became known as Brother Yun) reached innumerable people across China.

Along the way, Brother Yun married a young Chinese woman named Deling. She, too, had encountered God's unmistakable glory at a young age. In her childhood, Deling and her siblings worked long hours on their family farm, situated more than a mile from their home. The children had to walk to the fields in all weather, returning home each day with heavy loads of harvested cotton.

Deling suffered from hemophilia. That disease prevented her blood from clotting normally after an injury. Whenever she sustained a skin cut, which happened often in the cotton fields, the bleeding persisted for a long time. She wrapped her scraped feet and hands in rags to absorb the relentlessly oozing blood.

Deling's mother struggled with mental illness. While Deling was in her teens, her mother became a Christian. God then healed her mental illness. The whole family, indeed the whole village, soon noticed a major change in her mother's behaviour.

A neighbour told Deling that if she also committed her life to Christ, Jesus would heal her too. Eighteen-year-old Deling made that commitment. She began attending a local house church and soon after was baptized.

Days later, Deling had a vision in her sleep. In that vision, someone led her to dip her hands and feet in some clear water, and her scars disappeared. She awoke the next morning with her skin perfectly restored. She never again suffered from hemophilia.[15]

Deling married Brother Yun. Both remained motivated by what they had experienced in their youth and beyond: God's saving grace and His healing power. They couldn't stop speaking about His glory, no matter what it cost them personally. Willing to go anywhere and do anything, they suffered greatly. They pressed on, even after Brother Yun endured lengthy imprisonments and unspeakable torture. It comes as no surprise that signs and wonders, including many divine healings, accompanied their ministry. Deling has reported that healings commonly occurred, particularly during the explosion of church growth that occurred across China in the 1980s.[16]

The apostle Paul wrote, "… our gospel came to you not only in word, but also in power…" (1 Thessalonians 1:5a). Words are important, but God's power must be manifestly displayed so that our faith can be based on something more than an intellectual exercise. Our salvation and the spiritual transformation that occurs thereafter as we live out our Christian lives are two ways that God displays His glorious power. Healing is one more way in which God displays His power and His glory in our lives.

Some people believe it's selfish to pray for their own healing. If that resonates with you, I invite you to consider this: Maybe it's not all about you. Or me. It's partly about us, because our physical body and our health are involved. But it's not *all* about you or me. God wants to heal you to reveal His glory to you *and* to those around you. Could your healing be as much about Him and about others as it is about you? Be willing to let His glory shine through you. Just as Brother Yun and the rest of his family were drawn close to God by the healing of his father, perhaps your healing will draw others to God. The healing of Deling's mother brought Deling to faith in Christ and to her own healing.

Because healing brings God glory, we're compelled to do more than just seek healing. Let us remember to share our stories of healing. These stories bring Him glory every time they're told. King David wrote:

> *One generation shall commend your works to another, and*
> *shall declare your mighty acts. On the glorious splendor of your*
> *majesty, and on your wondrous works, I will meditate. They*
> *shall speak of the might of your awesome deeds, and I will declare*
> *your greatness. They shall pour forth the fame of your abundant*
> *goodness and shall sing aloud of your righteousness.*
>
> Psalm 145:4–7

May His glory be manifest in many ways around this world, including healing upon healing: your healing, my healing, and the healing of our loved ones. May we seek to glorify Him in response. When the time comes to leave this earth, may our attitude as we face death also bring Him glory. At that point, may we conduct ourselves as believers who eagerly anticipate coming into His glorious presence.

WHAT GOD EXPECTS US TO DO

7

ACCEPT HIS INVITATION

Years ago, I received an invitation to meet the Queen of England and other royal family members at a Buckingham Palace garden tea party. The invitation, embossed with fancy gilded letters, came in a large envelope with shiny gold lining inside. I had to formally accept the invitation. I later had to respect its terms: the time and date, the entrance gate I was to present at, the attire I had to wear, and some other protocols. I couldn't just show up at Buckingham Palace any time I wanted and expect to meet Queen Elizabeth on my own terms.

Let me tell you about a much more important royal invitation that has been sent to all of us. The King of kings and Lord of lords has invited us into *His* presence. He is extending *His* golden sceptre. He offers us infinitely more than tea, crumpets, and a brief one-time conversation. He invites us to be in an ongoing relationship with Him. He promises continuous access to His throne. We will never receive a better invitation than that.

God doesn't want us to merely know *about* Him. He wants us to *know* Him. We must, however, accept God's invitation on His own terms. Although I've been a Christian for decades, I still marvel that the Creator of the universe, God Almighty, wants to have a personal relationship with you and me.

Entering into a Relationship with God

We begin a relationship with God by responding to the invitation He has given regarding salvation through His Son, Jesus Christ. Unless we respond to that invitation, our sins will always separate us from God. The Bible tells us that we are *all* sinners who have fallen short of what God expects of us (Romans 3:23).

In Old Testament times, people made animal sacrifices to seek atonement for their sins. The New Testament tells us that God then provided a better way for humankind to be in right relationship with Him. God sent His only Son, Jesus, to this sin-wracked world to become the ultimate, permanent sacrifice. Jesus died on the cross as the *final* sacrifice for the sins of the world, including yours and mine.

If anyone confesses that they are a sinner, turns from all known wrongdoing, and asks for God's forgiveness (on the basis of what Jesus did), they enter into a personal relationship with God. Their sins will no longer separate them from Him. They can develop spiritual intimacy with Him. I have taken those steps, first as a six-year-old child, then with more mature understanding at age nineteen. I continue to freely admit that I am a sinner in need of a Saviour.

God is a triune God, one God comprising three persons. All those who have humbly knelt at the cross can enjoy rich fellowship with: God the Father; Jesus His risen Son (described in the Bible as our Saviour and Lord, but also our brother and friend); and the Spirit, who comes to indwell believers and wants to be our conscience, counsellor, comforter, and constant companion.

If you'd like to begin a personal relationship with God, you can turn to Appendix A, where you will find a prayer you can pray. If you're not sure whether you have accepted the gift of salvation in the past, I invite you to pray that prayer so that you *can* be sure that you are saved and in right standing with God. Don't entertain any doubt or uncertainty in this most important matter.

Maintaining Our Relationship with God

Once we enter into a relationship with God, we must try our best to avoid committing any further sins. We can learn the kinds of sins that bother God by getting to know the Bible, His Word. Thankfully, God doesn't expect us to be perfect. We all stumble and fall sometimes. God knows that we will still sin from time to time. Only Jesus walked without sin on this earth.

Every time we sin, we can confess that sin and repent of it to maintain ongoing right standing with God. Repentance means turning 180 degrees from the sinful attitude or activity. We're to deliberately travel in the opposite direction from whatever tempts us to sin. In response, God will forgive us and cleanse us from *all* sin (1 John 1:9). In God's eyes, it will be as if we had never sinned. He will wash us whiter than snow (Isaiah 1:18). We can go through this process of confession, repentance, and seeking His forgiveness over and over throughout our lifetimes.

Bible study is an important discipline that will help us draw closer to God. In His Word, God has revealed who He is, what He has done, what He requires of us, and what He plans to do in the future. I encourage you to read some portion of the Bible every day, even if you don't understand everything, even if you can only manage a few verses, even if you feel like you're fumbling around in the dark. His light will begin to dispel the darkness.

Prayer is another important daily discipline that can be developed.

I also encourage you to find a Bible-believing local church. The New Testament reveals many good reasons for belonging to a Christian community, including instruction from God's Word (and how it applies to our lives) and being prayed for.

The above activities will help us to develop and maintain a relationship with God. Let's seek to know the Healer before we seek His healing power.

Many Points of Access to God's Healing Power

In relationship with God, we have potential access to His healing power. Just as electric power can be accessed by many plug outlets and light switches in a home, God's healing power has many points of access through which it can flow. In my home, no electric power will be utilized until a light switch is turned on or an electrical cord is plugged in. There's constant potential for electric power to flow usefully through my home's wiring. Power will not actually flow, however, until it has been turned on or plugged into.

I can use a little electric power or a lot. It all depends on how many points of access I choose to implement. The power is ready to be used. The system is already in place. But the electric power is dormant until I deliberately activate it.

It's the same with God's healing power. Whether that power gets fully utilized in our lives depends to some extent on us. God supplies the power potential. It's up to us to access it. His Word tells us about the points of access through which His healing power can flow. That power doesn't automatically flow through every point. We have to *do* something at each point of access.

If we use one point of access, He might release some of His healing power. Why not use every point of access? The choice is ours. God will choose what measure of power He will release and the speed at which He releases it. I suspect that the number of access points that we activate will affect the measure and speed of healing, but, of course, God remains sovereign over the release of His power.

Jesus knew how to access God's power to heal. He taught His disciples how to access that power. When He sent the disciples out to preach and teach about the kingdom, He also sent them out to heal the sick. Training on how to access God's power to heal was passed on through the early centuries of the Christian church. Today, believers can access God's power to heal. We can learn how to use every point of access. You will encounter many such points in the pages to come.

A dry theology, based on mere words and doctrinal ideas, has limited value. God wants *His power to come down* to this earth. I love what Paul wrote in Ephesians 1:18–19: "Having the eyes of your hearts enlightened, that you may know… what is the immeasurable greatness of his [God's] power toward us who believe, according to the working of his [God's] great might…"

God wants to have His great power flow to us, in us, and through us to others. We must first individually respond to His royal invitation. We must enter into, and then maintain, a vital relationship with Him.

8

HONOUR OUR BODIES

Years ago, I attended a church service led by a well-known pastor in another city. At one point, congregants were welcomed to come forward for healing prayer. As people walked up the aisles, the pastor made a few comments to this effect: We cannot expect God to perform miracles with our health if we abuse or neglect our bodies.

Before considering how we might spiritually access God's healing power, let's consider how we treat our physical bodies. God designed our bodies to normally function well and to heal themselves, to some extent, when our health is impaired. We have to do everything we can to help with those processes. Certain laws of nature (ordained by God when He designed the human body) need to be respected.

We can partner with God in maintaining or restoring our health by taking reasonable care of our bodies. (It is, of course, more difficult to do so when we're sick, weak, and tired.) Wise self-care provides an important point of access to the immense healing power God has already programmed into our bodies.

Christians have at least five good motivations for taking care of their bodies:

1. God lovingly created us. Let's treat our bodies as valuable creations.

2. Jesus died for us. Paul wrote: "You are not your own; you were bought at a price. Therefore honor God with your bodies" (1 Corinthians 6:19b–20, NIV).

3. Our bodies are the temples in which the Holy Spirit resides (1 Corinthians 6:19). Consider how much God cared about the Temple in Jerusalem, a lifeless stone building made by human hands. Think about His detailed instructions regarding the maintenance of that Temple. Since the resurrection of Jesus, God has chosen for the Spirit to dwell within believers. How much more do you think God cares about the God-made temple of our living bodies?

4. Christians are called to be ambassadors for Christ (2 Corinthians 5:20). I've had the privilege of meeting many ambassadors. They're usually immaculately groomed and dressed, knowing they represent their nation. We represent the King of kings. Does the way we care for our bodies reflect that?

5. We'll likely optimize our health, strength, and energy if we maintain a wise lifestyle. We'll be better able to excel in the positions He has placed us in and to fulfil all the tasks He has appointed us. If we're always weak or weary, we're not likely to serve others well or be the best person we can be.

Three Key Elements

Nutrition, sleep, and exercise help us to maintain our best possible health, prevent illness, and restore compromised health.

Perhaps you're sick right now or recovering from injury or surgery. You may have little appetite. Maybe you cannot eat anything at all or are being fed intravenously. You might be bedridden and, ironically, not sleeping well. Perhaps you cannot walk much, if at all. You're welcome to skip this chapter if it feels burdensome at this present time.

You can always come back to it when your health has improved and you're better able to implement its principles.

Good Nutrition

So many clues to good nutrition can be found in the Bible. This should come as no surprise. Since God created our bodies in the first place, He has known all along what kinds of food will help them operate at their best.

God told Adam and Eve: "Behold, I have given you every plant yielding seed that is on the face of all the earth, and every tree with seed in its fruit. You shall have them for food" (Genesis 1:29). The human diet, at the very beginning, consisted of grains, vegetables, and fruits. Presumably, it also included the oils, nuts, spices, and herbs that plants produce.

In the garden, God didn't ordain heavy labour. Adam and Eve didn't need the calories, fat, and proteins that come from animal sources. It was only after they sinned that God told them they would have to get their food by the sweat of their brows, working in the field (Genesis 3:19). One of their sons, Abel, tended animal flocks (Genesis 4:2). Meat and dairy became part of their diet.

Some generations later, God told Noah and his sons:

> *The fear of you and the dread of you shall be upon every beast of the earth and upon every bird of the heavens, upon everything that creeps on the ground and all the fish of the seas. Into your hand they are delivered. Every moving thing that lives shall be food for you. And as I gave you the green plants, I give you everything.*
>
> Genesis 9:2–3

This added poultry, eggs, other birds, game, and fish to their diet. (Please note: When I use the word "diet," I do not mean a temporary diet designed to lose weight fast. I mean a regular dietary regimen, designed to promote good health over a lifetime, which becomes a lifestyle habit.)

Later in the Old Testament, we read about God placing some restrictions on what the Israelites could eat. For example, they weren't supposed to eat pork or shellfish. We won't review those restrictions, because Jesus removed them when He proclaimed that it's lawful to eat *all* things (Mark 7:14–19), restoring God's original permission to eat from the broad food groups described in Genesis. Food allergies, intolerances, and other health conditions might limit us, but otherwise, Jesus has granted us the freedom to eat whatever nutritious foods we enjoy. Peter later had a vision that reinforced the removal of the Old Testament distinction between what was "clean" to eat and what was "unclean" (Acts 10:9–16).

Let's look at what the Bible says about some specific food groups and then consider just a few of the good things we presently know about them.

Milk receives special status in the Bible. God referred to the Promised Land as the land of milk and honey (see, for example, Deuteronomy 31:20). We now know that milk provides fifteen essential nutrients, including calcium and magnesium (which benefit bones and teeth); protein (which builds/repairs various cells); vitamin A (important for vision and skin); vitamin B6, riboflavin, and zinc (which help to convert food into energy); vitamin B12 (necessary for red blood cell formation); thiamine (a promoter of overall growth); potassium (an aid to muscle and nerve function); and selenium (which benefits the immune system). Other dairy products, such as yogurt and cheese, provide many of those nutrients.

Bread also receives special biblical status. For example, the Lord's Prayer instructs us to ask for our daily bread (Matthew 6:11). Jesus referred to Himself as the Bread of Life (John 6:35). Jesus broke bread at the Last Supper and declared that bread would signify His crucified body in the sacrament of communion.

Bread provides important sustenance, yet many people shun bread these days instead of considering it a dietary staple. Like milk, bread usually contains calcium, magnesium, protein, vitamin B6, riboflavin, zinc, thiamine, potassium, and selenium. Bread might also contain iron (which helps to carry oxygen to cells); manganese (used to metabolise carbohydrates and cholesterol); and copper (necessary for iron metabolism and red blood cell formation). Bread provides carbohydrates (good for energy, mood elevation, heart health, and memory function) and fibre (which assists digestion). Grain-based pastas and cereals can also contribute to a healthy diet.

Not all grain products are equal. Highly processed white breads or pastas are not as healthy as whole-grain products. In biblical times, bread was simply made from wheat or barley, water, and salt. Contrast that with some of today's commercial products, which contain chemicals such as bleach and artificial preservatives. We can wisely assess the grains we consume.

Fruit receives favourable mention in the Bible. The Garden of Eden was full of fruit. The Promised Land offered abundant fruit. The spies who first went into that land found grapes, figs, and pomegranates (Numbers 13:23). People in biblical times also ate dates, apples, and olives. In the New Testament, fruit is an appealing metaphor for the good attributes of the Holy Spirit, such as love, joy, and peace (Galatians 5:22–23).

We now know that fruit has many nutritional assets, including fibre; vitamin C (an antioxidant that helps to produce collagen, brain neurotransmitters, and mood-regulating serotonin); potassium (which can help to lower blood pressure); and folate (a B vitamin that assists with cell division).

Vegetables are valued in the Bible. In biblical times, people ate vegetables such as beans, cucumbers, leeks, and onions. Esau wanted Jacob's red-lentil stew so much that he traded his birthright for that pot of vegetarian stew (Genesis 25:29–30). Daniel chose not to eat the royal food he was offered while serving in the king's palace. Instead, he (and other young Jewish men) requested a diet of vegetables and water (Daniel 1:12). After only ten days on that regimen, Daniel and the other three "… looked healthier and better nourished than any of the young men who ate the royal food" (Daniel 1:15, NIV). We now know that vegetarian or vegan diets, if properly structured, can be nutritionally sound.

Cruciferous vegetables (such as broccoli, cauliflower, and kale) are considered top cancer-fighting foods. Consumption of such vegetables has been shown to lower the risk of developing lung, bladder, breast, stomach, and colon cancers. Eating a broader range of vegetables (many colours of the rainbow) can lower the risk of developing heart disease, obesity, kidney stones, and type 2 diabetes. Vegetables contain many nutrients, such as folate, iron, potassium, and vitamins A and C.

Meat and **fish** are mentioned in the Bible. Lamb was mandated to be part of the Passover meal. In biblical times, people also ate beef, goat, and venison. Fish attains particular prominence in the New Testament. Jesus multiplied a few fish to feed thousands of people (Matthew 14:13–21). Jesus cooked fish for His disciples (John 21:9–13). Some of them were fishermen, so it's likely that Jesus ate fish often. I find it fascinating that the ancient symbol of a Christian believer was a fish. We now know that meat and fish contain protein and minerals, such as iron and zinc. (We also know that red meat and processed meat should be eaten in moderation.)

Oils are referred to in the Bible. Olive oil was the main oil consumed back then. Priests in the Old Testament were anointed with an oil mixture that included olive oil. In the New Testament, elders anointed people with a similar oil mixture before praying for their healing. Oil is one symbol of the Holy Spirit in scripture. Oil is currently used in certain church sacraments. We now know that olive oil is one of the healthiest oils to ingest, rich in anti-inflammatory, antioxidant power.

In contrast, Leviticus 7:22 prohibited eating the animal fat attached to meat. In recent decades, nutritionists have come to understand the health hazards of eating excess animal fat.

Nuts, seeds, spices, and **herbs** eaten in biblical times included almonds, pistachios, cumin, mustard, cinnamon, dill, garlic, and mint, which all have health benefits. Nuts are good sources of dietary fibre and nutrients, such as B group vitamins, vitamin E, calcium, iron, zinc, potassium, magnesium, selenium, and copper. Cinnamon has anti-inflammatory properties. Garlic contributes to heart health.

I encourage you to learn more about the nutritious value of various foods and to discover which foods might be helpful for your particular health concerns. Eating a variety of delicious foods can promote health, healing, strength, and energy.

The recommendations of modern First World governments regarding a healthy diet are remarkably in tune with the foods mentioned most favourably and prominently in the Bible. Current recommendations include eating whole-grain products, an abundance of fruit and vegetables (preferably fresh), milk products (preferably low-fat), lean meats, fish, "good" oils (such as olive oil), nuts, and seeds. A dietary regimen based on foods native to the Mediterranean area (similar to what Jesus and His disciples probably ate) now ranks as one of the healthiest diets.

Current nutritional guides also advise that we should add minimal salt and processed sugar to our food and watch out for "bad" fats, such as trans-fat or partially hydrogenated fat. Salt, sugar, and "bad" fats are well known to harm our health if consumed in excess.

Speaking of excess, we all know that we should maintain a healthy weight. This is certainly a challenge, especially as we get older. We can joke about the extra pounds we carry, but the fact that more than one billion people in our world are considered obese is not a laughing matter. Obesity carries with it a wide range of health risks. I invite you to research the number of servings (and portion sizes) you should have of each food group each day, depending on your age, sex, and health status.

The best foods we can eat (for nutritional content *and* reasonable calorie count) come straight from nature, in the original state in which God created them, altered as little as possible by human processing. God has richly deposited His life-sustaining power in the vitamins, minerals, proteins, carbohydrates, phytochemicals, fibres, and other good components of the whole foods that He has created for our benefit.

If only we could grow all of our vegetables in our own gardens, pick fruit from our own orchards, harvest our own grain, milk our own cow, catch our own fish, and collect our own eggs! It's not realistic, however, for most of us to do that. We must make wise choices in a grocery store. We can choose products that are as fresh and unprocessed as possible. Canned or frozen foods can be good choices if they have limited salt, sugar, and chemical additives.

I don't do any of this perfectly. I confess that I have a weakness for potato chips and other not-so-healthy foods. I buy some prepackaged convenience foods. I suspect many of you can relate. I try to eat healthy foods most of the time but allow myself limited indulgences. As with every other area of life, God knows we won't be perfect. If we confess our mistakes, God will help us to start afresh each day, to eat as best we can.

Whenever we do buy something highly processed, loaded with salt or sugar, we can add as many natural ingredients as possible. For example, we can add chopped fresh vegetables to watered-down canned soup, or fresh meat to packaged rice mixes.

Some people stress about environmental contaminants. Many toxins in air, soil, and water end up in our food and drink. Fresh fruits and vegetables, for example, might arrive in our grocery store loaded with pesticides. Foods that have passed through processing factories (even fresh salad greens) can be tainted with salmonella or listeria. We must ask for God's protection over our food and drink. Exodus 23:25 promises that He will bless the bread and water of those who obey Him. That verse supports the Judeo-Christian practice of praying a blessing over meals before partaking.

Mark 16:18 states: "… if they [believers] drink any deadly poison, it will not hurt them…" I trust, on the basis of that verse, that chemicals, bad bacteria, and other foreign molecules in our food and drink will not unduly harm us.

Let's not stress about our food and drink. We must accept that not all produce gets grown organically and locally. Not all meat comes from animals grown free-range, or without antibiotics and added hormones. We may have budgetary constraints that do not permit us to always buy fresh food. We may have time constraints that don't permit us to cook from scratch very often. Let's not go overboard and make imperfect food our enemy. God wants us to enjoy our food and drink. Many verses discuss that in the book of Ecclesiastes. We can apply the best wisdom and knowledge of which we're aware, thank God for our imperfect meals, and pray for His grace and blessing over them.

"Oh, taste and see that the Lord is good!" (Psalm 34:8a). Applied literally, we can experience God's goodness while tasting the wide array of nutritious, delicious foods He has designed and created for us.

Sleep and Rest

In our modern world, getting enough sleep is a real challenge. In many careers, workers are expected to burn the midnight oil. People also stay up late surfing the Internet, watching TV, or finishing domestic chores.

If we ignore our need for sleep, we will eventually pay a price. Our bodies *need* sleep to repair and replace cells, to fight viruses and infections, and to simply recharge. God wants to give us sleep (Psalm 127:2), but we have to do our part to facilitate it.

The most obvious way to get more sleep is to routinely go to bed earlier. We can also sleep better if we:

- limit caffeine, especially late in the day
- avoid or limit alcohol intake
- avoid eating or exercising in the few hours before bedtime (although exercising earlier in the day helps induce deep sleep)
- invest in the best quality mattresses and pillows that we can afford
- avoid electronic devices late at night
- enjoy a warm bath before bed
- sleep in a dark, quiet room in a comfortable temperature (different for everyone and changing as we age)
- do anything else we have found to be sleep-inducing (experiment with what works best for you)

Optimal sleep duration for most people clocks in at about seven or eight hours. Too much or too little sleep isn't good for us.

If we're really sleep deprived, we can seek medication as short-term therapy to help us get back into a good sleeping pattern. Sleeping pills can be a blessing, but they aren't meant to be a permanent aid. Those who suffer chronic insomnia can undergo a sleep study and seek medical help for sleep disorders, such as apnea.

Anxiety, depression, anger, and stress can interfere with sleep. We can seek remedies for those conditions, too, including medication and/or counselling. We can also ask God to provide sleep and to help us manage our thoughts and feelings while we wait to fall asleep or if we wake up in the middle of the night.

I once read that some Christians, in medieval times, routinely prayed in the middle of the night. They went to bed when darkness fell and would often be there for ten or twelve hours. They might sleep for four hours, then be awake for a few hours, and then sleep again. Some considered their nocturnal waking hours the perfect time to commune with God, when the world around them was quiet and still. Children were sleeping, no duties or distractions beckoned. This became a natural and accepted rhythm of life, greeted with peace and joy (instead of the stress we often feel if we toss and turn at two o'clock in the morning). The next time you're awake in the wee hours, consider spending time with God.

I sometimes wake up during the night. If I think about hurts or troubles, I might be up for hours. I pray in those dark hours, but not in great detail about pain or problems. I've learned (the hard way) that it's better to pray about tough issues when I'm awake the next day. In the night, I focus on thanking God for specific blessings and praising Him for His wonderful qualities. I might also mentally sing a worship song that invokes calm and comfort. Disciplining my mind to think and pray only positive thoughts helps me drift back to sleep.

And what about rest during the day? God commanded us to rest one day every week: "Six days shall work be done, but the seventh day is a Sabbath of solemn rest, holy to the Lord" (Exodus 31:15a). Even God worked for six days and then, on the seventh day, He did not work. He was "rested" and "refreshed" on that day (v. 17). In early Christianity, the Sabbath was considered to be Saturday; today, it's usually celebrated on Sundays. Your job might not permit you to take every Sunday off work (for example, if you are a pastor, an emergency physician, a police officer, or a firefighter). In that case, find a weekday to rest.

Every day, we can seek some moments of rest. In Mark 6:31, Jesus told His disciples to "rest a while" in a desolate place. (They did not succeed in getting away from the crowds on that occasion, but Jesus likely repeated the suggestion.)

The need for rest is programmed into the human body. Our ears, for example, need to regularly rest. Music with lots of rest notes is easy to listen to, whether it is soothing or stirring. Music without rest notes creates non-stop noise, an assault to the brain. Our ears and our minds tire quickly if there are no pauses.

Similarly, our eyes need to rest when we read. Written sentences are supposed to end with a period so our eyes and mind can rest every line or two. A well-known author, James Joyce, wrote a book called *Ulysses*. One section of it, called Molly Bloom's soliloquy, consists of two supersized sentences. The first sentence drags on for 11,281 words. The second contains 12,931 words. Imagine two sentences galloping for about sixty pages without periods. When I read that soliloquy in university, my head ached from the visual and mental stress. I felt cross-eyed by the end of it! The stream of words eventually became gibberish to me, because the missing punctuation had not permitted my eyes and my mind to enjoy frequent rest stops.

I encourage you to find daily moments to rest, along with one day a week of rest, and seasonal periods of rest, such as vacations or staycations.

Exercise

God designed our bodies to benefit from daily exercise. Jesus and His disciples led a physically active life. They walked everywhere, travelling between villages on foot, carrying whatever they needed. If they had step trackers, they would likely have logged tens of thousands of steps most days. They walked uphill and downhill in places such as Jerusalem, Judea, and Galilee. They didn't need a gym step machine. When they crossed the Sea of Galilee, they didn't relax while a crew manned the ship. *They* had to man the sails and use the oars. *They* had to haul in fishing nets. Back on shore, *they* had to collect firewood and then cook their fish dinners.

The apostle Paul wrote: "…train yourself for godliness; for while bodily training is of some value, godliness is of value in every way, as it holds promise for the present life and also for the life to come" (1 Timothy 4:7–8). Paul didn't say that exercise was a total waste of time. He conceded that physical exercise provides *some* benefit. His point was that our spiritual life takes *precedence* over physical exercise, but spirituality does not remove the need for daily exercise.

Paul's words might convict someone who spends mega-hours at the gym, or every weekend playing sports, but who doesn't spend much (if any) time praying, reading the Bible, or attending church. At the other extreme, Paul's words should *not* be used as an excuse to avoid exercise. Most of us are too sedentary. Many of us live in suburbs, drive most places, work on computers, and watch some television. Sitting too much jeopardizes our health. Some doctors even say that sitting is the new smoking.

Perhaps you can't afford a gym membership, special sports clothing, or expensive athletic equipment. Plain old-fashioned walking works wonders. One half-hour of brisk walking each day provides many health benefits. That half-hour can be broken down into two fifteen-minute sessions or three ten-minute sessions, if necessary. We can also do housework and yard work with gusto, counting those tasks as exercise.

I can think of at least a dozen good reasons to exercise. It:

- helps us to achieve (and maintain) a healthy weight
- elevates our mood
- alleviates anxiety and depression
- strengthens muscles, joints, tendons, ligaments, and bones
- gives our heart and lungs a workout
- boosts energy
- kicks our calorie-burning metabolism into higher gear
- improves our body image and appearance
- stimulates digestion and circulation
- boosts brain function
- makes our skin glow
- sometimes gets us outdoors in fresh air, sunshine, and nature
- sometimes facilitates social time with family and friends

Let's get motivated and get moving!

Stress Management

Some have grown accustomed to thinking of stress as a purely negative force. We might stress about our stress. That's not helpful. Not all stress is negative. Short-lived stress helps us to deal effectively with a sudden crisis. Stress can create energy and focus. Acute stress can positively help us with activities such as studying for an exam and then writing it. Stress can help us to do many other things with all pistons firing. Successful people have learned to see *some* measure of stress as their friend, not their enemy.

Constant long-term stress, on the other hand, can damage our health and rob us of energy. That's when stress becomes debilitating. Healthy living can help to manage our stress. Research has shown that adequate sleep, nutrition, and exercise all fuel positive stress and mediate negative stress.

Taking Care of Ourselves When Caregiving

Perhaps a loved one is sick, injured, or recovering from surgery. Perhaps you're an exhausted, depleted caregiver. I encourage you to take whatever time and effort is necessary to take care of your *own* self.

When my husband was in the hospital for a while, a nurse encouraged me to play my usual midweek tennis game. She told me not to feel guilty or selfish leaving the ICU for a few hours. The games I played those weeks were hyper-adrenaline-driven games. I hammered the tennis balls across the net. I played better than ever because, with each hit, I was releasing so much bottled-up stress. I strengthened myself for the marathon of caregiving that lay ahead in my husband's recovery-at-home phase.

Take care to eat well. Keep hydrated. Get out in the fresh air for a walk. Find moments of rest and refreshment. I've done this during many hospitalizations of loved ones. It has helped me to be a better caregiver in the long run.

God Won't Honour Our Neglect of Our Health

Young people often enjoy good health and might feel invincible, but sooner or later, we all realize that we're far from invincible. Once health issues arise, God won't likely heal our bodies if we don't routinely honour them. We must accept responsibility for our health.

If we haven't been wise in the past, we can ask God to forgive our foolish ways. We don't have to get stuck in guilt, regret, or shame. We can ask for His help moving onward. Perhaps you've lived on junk food or have been a couch potato. Maybe you've abused drugs, alcohol, or cigarettes. Perhaps you've been injured while engaging in a risky activity. Even if you bear some blame for your health issue, God can extend mercy if you want a fresh start. While He may allow us to suffer some consequences from imprudent decisions, He longs to help us change our ways. This moment begins the rest of your life. If need be, ask God to forgive the past and help you develop a better lifestyle and become a good steward of your body.

Beyond Honouring Our Bodies

While wise health habits will certainly benefit us, they aren't enough to ensure constant good health. No matter how disciplined we are, we don't have complete control over our health. That's why there are still many chapters to read! Let's move on to discuss spiritual practices relating to health and healing. We can take many steps to invite Him (the one who *is* in control) and His power into our health situation.

9

KNOW GOD'S WORD

A few decades ago, two serious and unexpected hospitalizations occurred. My dad suffered back-to-back massive heart attacks. Two months later, another close family member suddenly developed a major health issue.

Looking back, God had prepared me for that stressful season in an interesting way. Months prior, I'd been challenged by a retreat speaker to begin collecting Bible verses that would inspire God-focused hope in future times of crisis. She gave each woman a notebook in which we could start writing down verses. Numerous pages in my notebook soon filled up. I loved my daily quest for *more* verses. Most evenings, as I prepared dinner, I propped my notebook up on a recipe book stand and meditated on my accumulated verses, letting them sink deep into my spirit.

During the later hospitalizations of my two family members, I carried that notebook around with me every day. The verses scribed within it grounded me, providing hope, along with peace, strength, faith, and comfort. I read them over and over, memorizing many of them.

Wonderful as my broad collection of verses was, I decided to begin a new collection, concentrating on healing. I typed out every verse I could find. That compilation has been of great importance during subsequent illnesses, injuries, and hospitalizations. That second collection has provided a solid foundation for this book.

God's Word offers us a *key* point of access to His healing power. Proverbs 4:20–22 declares:

> *My child, pay attention to what I say. Listen carefully to my words. Don't lose sight of them. Let them penetrate deep into your heart, for they bring life to those who find them, and healing to their whole body.* (NLT)

Do you want life? Do you want healing for your whole body? Then listen to God's words (at *least* as diligently as you listen to what doctors say about your health). Do not lose sight of God's words. We should spend more time looking at His words than at our physical symptoms. Staring at an ugly rash, a pink eye, or a festering sore won't make such conditions go away.

God's words generate life and promote health. They can impact every cell in our bodies. We can take in His words every day as faithfully as we take prescribed medication. Medication usually targets one area of the body, such as an arthritic joint or a sinus infection. God's Word can saturate the entire body with its life-enhancing power.

Reading the Bible will keep us very close to God. Some people say that they go through times when He seems far away. God is *never* far away from anyone with access to His Word. If you feel that God is distant, or unreachable, I invite you to go to His Word. Immerse yourself in it. God is not silent. He constantly speaks through His Word. He encourages and comforts through His Word. The Bible can invigorate and revive us. It can teach us everything we need to know about God.

Here's an astonishing fact: Jesus, the Son of God, *is* the Word (John 1:1). When we know, love, revere, and rely on the Bible, we are also knowing, loving, revering, and relying on Jesus. Those who truly grasp that Jesus *is* the Word will surely read, memorize, and utilize the Word of God with greater passion and purpose.

No wonder Hebrews 4:12 declares that the Word is "living and active." It embodies the living power of the risen Christ. Let's allow God's words to be alive and active within our physical bodies (and, indeed, within our entire lives). In 1 Corinthians 4:20, we learn that the kingdom of God does not just come to us with God's words, but also with God's power. Healing power flows through some of God's words.

Jesus compared divine words to seeds (see, for example, the parable of the sower in Matthew 13). Such seeds will bear fruit if planted in a receptive, fertile heart. We can plant word-seeds in our own hearts.

While Jesus was on earth, His spoken words healed people, if the hearers believed His words. John 4:46b–53a, for example, presents this story:

> ... *at Capernaum there was an official whose son was ill. When this man heard that Jesus had come from Judea to Galilee, he went to him and asked him to come down and heal his son, for he was at the point of death. So Jesus said to him, "Unless you see signs and wonders you will not believe." The official said to him, "Sir, come down before my child dies." Jesus said to him, "Go; your son will live." The man believed the word that Jesus spoke to him and went on his way. As he was going down, his servants met him and told him that his son was recovering. So he asked them the hour when he began to get better, and they said to him, "Yesterday at the seventh hour the fever left him." The father knew that was the hour when Jesus had said to him, "Your son will live."*

When the official asked Jesus to heal his son, Jesus accused the man of wanting to see a miracle before he believed. Despite this rebuke, the father unflinchingly repeated his request. Jesus saw that the man already had belief that He could heal. Jesus declared to the man that his son would live. The "man *believed the word* that Jesus spoke to him and went on his way" (v. 50b). The father no longer begged Jesus to travel some distance to his son's bedside. The word of Jesus was enough. Today, the Word of Jesus is still enough.

Jesus healed by words alone on many other occasions. In Matthew 8:5–13, we find this story:

> *When he [Jesus] had entered Capernaum, a centurion came*
> *forward to him, appealing to him, "Lord, my servant is lying*
> *paralyzed at home, suffering terribly." And he [Jesus] said to him,*
> *"I will come and heal him." But the centurion replied, "Lord, I*
> *am not worthy to have you come under my roof, but only say the*
> *word, and my servant will be healed. For I too am a man under*
> *authority, with soldiers under me. And I say to one, 'Go,' and he*
> *goes, and to another, 'Come,' and he comes, and to my servant,*
> *'Do this,' and he does it." When Jesus heard this, he marveled and*
> *said to those who followed him, "Truly, I tell you, with no one in*
> *Israel have I found such faith…" And to the centurion Jesus said,*
> *"Go; let it be done for you as you have believed." And the servant*
> *was healed at that very moment.*

Like the official in the first story, the Roman centurion knew that the words of Jesus contained sufficient authority and power to heal.

On other occasions, Jesus spoke directly to the person in need. Some friends or relatives brought a paralyzed man, lying on a mat, to Jesus: "… He [Jesus] said to the paralyzed man, 'Get up, take your mat and go home.' Then the man got up and went home" (Matthew 9:6b–7, NIV). The paralytic, believing the words of Jesus, was empowered to rise up and start walking. He walked all the way back home.

Another time, Jesus visited the Pool of Bethesda in Jerusalem (a place you can still visit today). A man who had been an invalid for thirty-eight years was lying down by the water. Other people with disabilities surrounded the pool, believing that its water contained special healing properties. After the invalid explained his frustration about trying to get down into the water, Jesus said: "Get up! Pick up your mat and walk" (John 5:8). The invalid obeyed Him and was instantly healed (John 5:9). He didn't need the special water after all. Jesus later found the man in the nearby temple, still walking and well.

Yes, power permeates the words of Jesus—not just the spoken words of Jesus from two millennia ago, but also the *whole* Word of God, which we have established *is* Jesus. Through the Bible, Jesus can speak to you and to me this very hour, wherever we are. Jesus longs to speak to us.

Faith comes from hearing the Word of God (Romans 10:17). When we encounter His words and choose to believe them, faith arises in us, as it did in the four men just mentioned. We cannot have true faith without knowing God's Word. Authentic Christian faith is always based *on* the Word; otherwise, our faith is based on something less (wishful thinking, our own desire, man's medicine, or seeing improvement of symptoms). Knowledge of the Bible must *precede* the acquisition of true faith.

The early Christians grasped the power of the Word and its direct link to healing. Peter prayed: "And now… grant to your servants to continue to *speak your word* with all boldness, while you [the Lord] stretch out your hand to heal, and signs and wonders are performed through the name of your holy servant Jesus" (Acts 4:29–30). First-century Christians believed that their Lord would stretch out His divine hand to heal as they proclaimed His Word.

Jesus wants us to discover the power of His Word. He declared: "If you abide in me [Jesus], and my *words* abide in you, ask whatever you wish, and it will be done for you" (John 15:7). How willing are you to receive God's words, to believe them, and perhaps this very hour to stake your life on them? Sadly, not every Christian will answer in the affirmative.

I used to offer my collection of healing-related verses to any Christian who told me they were dealing with a health issue. It surprised me that not everyone appreciated that gesture. Some were resistant to receiving those verses. The more I've grown to understand the theology of certain churches, the more I understand the cool reaction. Some churches teach that after the deaths of Jesus and the early apostles, God stopped offering believers access to His healing power. They consider the healing stories in the Bible as nothing more than ancient history.

I've also been surprised to discover how biblically illiterate many Christians are today. In 2013, the Canadian Bible Forum (nine Bible agencies and The Evangelical Fellowship of Canada) engaged a market research company, Angus Reid, to undertake the Canadian Bible Engagement Study. Angus Reid interviewed more than 4,500 people, making the study the most comprehensive national study of its kind. It revealed many details about Bible reading, with the overall finding being that most Canadians are *not* reading the Bible. Between 1996 and 2013, Bible reading declined by 60 percent. In 2013, only 14 percent of Christians perused their Bible at least once a month.[17]

The study further revealed that many Canadians no longer believe that the Bible is the Word of God. Even some Christians question the trustworthiness of the Bible and do not equate it with truth. We're surrounded by a culture that denies the existence of absolute truth. Our Western culture asserts that you can have your truth, and I can have a different truth, and no one can claim to possess timeless, universal truth.

If Christian faith comes from the Word of God, how strong can a person's faith be if they don't know the Word, or even want to know the Word? And on what exactly are they basing their faith if it's not God's Word?

I am thoroughly convinced that the Bible is the Word of God. I know I'm not alone. Many friends and family members, some of them highly educated in academic and professional disciplines, also believe that the Bible is the true, timeless, and only Word of God. If you're not convinced of this, I encourage you to find books that examine and defend the authenticity and reliability of the Bible as God's revealed Word. You must choose what you will believe about the Bible. If you don't believe that it's the true and trustworthy Word of God, this book will be of limited value to you.

Some Stories

In my mid-twenties, while travelling through India, I experienced days of high fever alternating with severe, body-wracking chills. Becoming too sick to leave my hotel room, I lay on the bed beneath a slowly turning ceiling fan. The fan cooled me during dramatic fever spikes. Then, when my body temperature dipped, I shivered and shook uncontrollably. I piled mounds of clothing on myself to keep warm. Each time the fever spiked, my body fired up anew, and I threw off the pile of clothes. My head hurt continuously. My whole body ached from the violent spells of shaking, shivering, and sweating profusely. At times, I struggled to breathe normally. Fatigue overwhelmed me. I could barely pray.

My sister became concerned enough to visit a pharmacist at a five-star hotel. He suspected that I had malaria, a serious disease and potentially fatal if left untreated. He gave her chloroquine pills (a drug treatment that was effective back in the 1970s, before mosquitoes became resistant to it). My symptoms began abating while taking the pills.

Back in Canada, three months after the fever-and-chills attack, my hair began to fall out. At first, I noticed many strands in the sink after a hair wash. Then a more alarming amount of fallen hair tangled up in the teeth of my comb and the bristles of my hairbrush. I marvelled that I had any hair left on my head.

My hair continued to fall out over the next few weeks. It was a miracle of sorts that my thinning hair didn't look worse than it did. I consulted the best hair stylist in the city. He cut my hair shorter. While blow-drying my hair, he commented that the clumps gathering in his brush rivalled the hair loss of cancer patients undergoing active treatment. He grimly predicted that I would lose all of my hair by month's end if I continued to lose strands at that rate.

I sought medical help. The first specialist, an expert in tropical disease, told me I had likely suffered from either malaria or scarlet fever in India. He couldn't guarantee that my hair would grow back. If scarlet fever had been the culprit, my hair loss might be permanent. You can imagine my shock and fear.

That doctor passed my case along to a dermatologist who specialized in hair follicle issues. She did some tests and concluded that I had contracted malaria in India. My hair loss was a temporary after-effect of the fever spells. The good news: Most likely my hair would eventually grow back. The bad news: It would probably all fall out first. I cried while stumbling down the stairs of the subway station soon after. This might surprise those who know me well, because I don't cry often. I had just started my year as an articling student in a big city law firm. The prospect of being bald for a while horrified me.

I began reading my Bible more than usual. On one particularly discouraging day, these verses comforted me:

> *But now, this is what the Lord says—he who created you… he who formed you… "Do not fear, for I have redeemed you; I have summoned you by name; you are mine. When you pass through the waters, I will be with you; and when you pass through the rivers, they will not sweep over you. When you walk through the fire, you will not be burned; the flames will not set you ablaze."*
>
> Isaiah 43:1–2, NIV

Those words assured me that, although I would go through difficult circumstances, all would be well in the end. Although those verses weren't about healing, they still imparted faith that I would be healed.

I was also comforted by Jesus' words in this one simple sentence: "… even the hairs of your head are all numbered…" (Luke 12:7a). Jesus counted every single hair that fell from my head. He knew how many still remained. He knew when my hair would start to grow back. He cared *that* intimately about my situation. Nine words helped me believe that the same God who had healed the malaria could stop and reverse the disturbing hair loss. My abnormal hair loss ended abruptly one day, and my hair was rapidly restored to normal volume.

On another occasion, God highlighted a specific verse in my inner spirit. After our young adult son underwent abdominal surgery, the lead surgeon advised us that it had been successful. No complications had occurred. The first post-op days went remarkably smoothly. Discharge from the hospital seemed in sight.

While our son napped one afternoon, I went out for a walk. On that spring day, crocuses and tulips colourfully bloomed, and lime-green leaf buds brightened every tree branch. The city streets teemed with cheerful-yellow taxis. I prayed as I walked, sang to myself, and praised God, expressing gratitude that our son seemed to be doing well.

While walking, Psalm 23 came to mind. My memory reviewed the whole Psalm. (It's helpful to have God's Word buried deep within us. We can readily retrieve it, summoning it at will. Other times, the Spirit might cause stored verses to bubble up into our conscious mind when we most need them.) As my mind journeyed through Psalm 23, verse two (about green pastures and serene waters) resonated with my mood. It felt compatible with the warm sunshine, the greening grass, the blue skies, and the joyful birdsong.

The Spirit did not let me linger on the idyllic scene in verse two. Instead, I felt an inner shift of focus to verse four: "Even though I walk through the valley of the shadow of death, I will fear no evil, for you are with me; your rod and your staff, they comfort me."

I did not *want* to focus on verse four. The inner prompting to think about a dark valley, or the nearness of death, seemed strange. My son wasn't dying. He was recovering well. Perhaps, I told myself, it wasn't the Spirit nudging my thoughts. When I tried to eject verse four from my mind, but couldn't, I somehow knew that the strong emphasis on that verse came from the Spirit.

Later that evening, my son's seemingly great recovery unravelled quickly. He developed a high fever and an elevated heart rate. His belly became hard. He complained of increasingly severe abdominal pain. He felt exhausted and looked jaundiced. Those symptoms escalated on the following day, Easter Sunday. Only a skeletal staff remained in the hospital. The junior resident on duty didn't want to call in the senior resident, let alone the staff surgeon. My husband, a doctor, kept insisting on an immediate abdominal tap to obtain a sample of the fluid that was clearly accumulating in our son's belly. Finally, the senior surgeon was called at home. He agreed that the tap procedure should be done immediately, along with some other tests.

After the results came in, our son was rushed into emergency surgery. We learned that his small bowel had perforated (probably caused by post-surgical blood clots pressing against the bowel). A massive amount of toxins had spilled into his abdomen. The surgical team had to clean out the abdominal cavity to reduce the level of infection. Our son remained in critical condition, however, because a life-threatening amount of infection had already invaded his bloodstream. After hours of surgery, our son was moved to the ICU.

During my shell-shocked, gut-wrenching drive home, verse four of Psalm 23 came back to me. This time the verse about the dark valley didn't seem so grim. In fact, it actually uplifted me. Deep within, the Spirit impressed upon me that my son was just *passing through* the valley of the *shadow* of death. We would only encounter death's dark shadow, but not actual death. The valley would indeed be dark and dangerous, but I sensed that we would emerge on the other side in a much better place, just as David did by the end of Psalm 23. And God would be our Shepherd along the way. I felt comfort and assurance. I could press on praying with faith.

That verse, along with countless others, sustained me through what became a difficult forty-day hospitalization (mostly spent in the step-down ICU). I sometimes prayed out loud beside our son's bed, quoting verses, even when our son slept or was heavily sedated by pain medication. Not knowing if he heard my prayers, or the verses I quoted, I kept praying out loud anyway. I believed that the words of God never return to Him void of effect; His words always accomplish the purposes for which they were sent (Isaiah 55:11). I pled with God for my son's healing on the basis of His own words.

At first, I felt self-conscious praying out loud, quoting verses about healing, but I believed in the power that the proclaimed living Word releases. It benefitted my own soul to hear God's words spoken out loud.

I encourage you to declare God's words over sick loved ones. You might feel foolish. You might fear that a doctor will come into the room. Perhaps you might even fear what your family members will think. When my son was in the hospital, I worried that if he wasn't healed, he'd abandon his faith. Even though I often felt both foolish and fearful when I prayed God's words out loud (especially when not much improvement seemed to be happening), I chose to persist. I believed God's words would impact the situation.

Peter asked God for boldness to speak His Word and for God to stretch forth His hand to heal (Acts 4:29–30). We, too, must be ready to speak His Word boldly when we ask God to extend His healing hand.

I marvel at the great measure of healing that God eventually granted our son. The medical team had told us that there were grave limits to what they could do during our son's struggle. God's wonder-working power did the rest.

I reminded myself of the Word's power when my husband, Sam, was suddenly hospitalized because of a brain bleed. I've already explained that during the massive hemorrhaging, Sam's brain was in great danger. He was concurrently in stage-four heart failure and close to renal failure because of the extent to which his kidneys began malfunctioning.

One of the first verses I quoted to myself, and to Sam, was John 10:10: "The thief comes only to steal and to kill and to destroy. I [Jesus] came that they may have life and have it abundantly." I held on to that verse like one would grab on to a branch overhead if thrashing in a river about to spill over a waterfall. Every time I felt panic, I meditated on that verse.

I was concerned about Sam's life but also about his full recovery. I knew the serious damage he could suffer if the growing pool of blood accumulating in the hollow centre of his brain began penetrating surrounding brain tissue. At the point of diagnosis, the mass of blood already pressed dangerously against that tissue. I didn't want Sam to merely live; I wanted him to *fully* live again.

Another Bible passage that bubbled up into my mind was Philippians 4:6–7: "Do not be anxious about anything, but in every situation, by prayer and petition, with thanksgiving, present your requests to God. And the peace of God, which transcends all understanding, will guard your hearts and your minds in Christ Jesus" (NIV). That final clause primarily refers to Christ guarding our feelings and thoughts, but I believe it can also refer to Him guarding our *physical* hearts and minds.

As I prayed those verses over Sam, I asked God to guard Sam's heart and mind on both levels as he began to comprehend his critical condition. I asked God to guard my own heart and mind.

This verse also came to me: "For God has not given us a spirit of fear, but of power and of love and of a sound mind" (2 Timothy 1:7, NKJV). I asked God to protect Sam's mind.

I had a dozen typed pages of other applicable verses with me at the hospital, and I spoke and prayed those over Sam too. One wonderful by-product of my focus on the Word: I felt that God (the Father, Jesus, and the Spirit) was very close by and that, indeed, the Spirit was within me. I cannot emphasize enough that when we focus on the Word, we're hearing the voice of Jesus because He *is* the Word. We're in communion with Him every time we partake of His Word, whether we're reading it on a printed page (or a digital page), hearing it, or thinking about it.

When I prayed verses out loud, Sam would open both hands and hold them upward, gesturing to God that he believed His Word and wanted to receive His healing power. I kept filling Sam's mind with God's words because I knew he needed them even more than I did. I didn't care if any of the nurses, serially posted at a desk right outside his room in the ICU, could hear what I was doing. I only cared that God could hear me and that Sam could (if awake) hear me too.

Such verses sustained Sam and me as he went through months of recovery. God gradually granted him a great measure of healing, and our lives have carried on over the years. We know that our united belief in God's Word supplied one crucial point of access to God's mighty healing power.

I've learned lessons from others about the importance of knowing, speaking, and praying God's words during a health struggle. Dodie, the mother of an American pastor I've met a few times, has demonstrated a Word-focused response to disease.

After weeks of fever, fatigue, insomnia, jaundice, and pain, Dodie sought medical advice. She was diagnosed in December 1981 with metastatic liver cancer. Pathologists, radiologists, and internists agreed upon the diagnosis, based upon a variety of tests, including a CT scan, a liver biopsy, and blood work. Her liver hosted a few tumours, one of them already the size of an orange. One doctor told Dodie that the cancer was so advanced, she likely had only a few weeks left to live.

Instead of starting chemotherapy, Dodie chose to rest at home over the Christmas season. Her doctor had opined that chemotherapy would not likely add much time to the short weeks she had remaining. (Cancer treatment was not as advanced back in 1981 as it is today.)

Dodie was initially shocked and then afraid, as anyone might be, with that grim diagnosis and prognosis. She was only forty-eight years old, with some of her five children still in their teens. Fear plagued her.

She looked in the bathroom mirror each morning and saw a haggard, yellowed, thinning face staring back. Her whole body became increasingly frail. Her weight dwindled as low as eighty-nine pounds.

She searched for Bible verses she could focus on. Psalm 118:17 became one of her favourites: "I shall not die, but I shall live, and recount the deeds of the Lord." She spoke that verse aloud as she shuffled around her house. It helped to offset five ominous words that echoed in her brain—"a few weeks to live."

Dodie chose to believe that she would live much longer than a few weeks. She relied on this passage:

> I [the Lord, through His spokesperson Moses] call heaven and earth
> to witness against you today, that I have set before you life and
> death, blessing and curse. Therefore choose life, that you and your
> offspring may live, loving the Lord your God, obeying his voice and
> holding fast to him, for he is your life and length of days...
>
> Deuteronomy 30:19–20a

Dodie asked God to do for her what He did for King Hezekiah back in Old Testament days. God had granted King Hezekiah the extra fifteen years he had prayed for. Instead of asking for fifteen, she boldly asked for twenty-five or thirty more years.

When friends asked about her condition, she replied, "By the stripes of Jesus, I'm healed" (from 1 Peter 2:24). She knew the principle, spelled out in Proverbs 18:21, that death and life are impacted by the tongue. Proverbs 10:11a states: "The mouth of the righteous is a fountain of life." Proverbs 14:3b asserts: "… the lips of the wise will preserve them." Instead of complaining about her cancer, she used her tongue to declare God's words.

Dodie meditated on many other scripture verses and often declared them aloud. Her husband, a pastor, spoke verses to her and over her. They had united faith in the Bible and what it said about healing. Years before, they had prayed together, and believed in God's Word together, for the healing of their baby daughter, born with a condition similar to cerebral palsy. God had performed a miracle in their tiny daughter, who grew up to be physically normal.

Dodie chose to believe that Psalm 91:14–16 applied to her:

> *The Lord says, "I will rescue those who love me. I will protect*
> *those who trust in my name. When they call on me, I will answer;*
> *I will be with them in trouble. I will rescue and honor them. I will*
> *reward them with a long life and give them my salvation." (NLT)*

Dodie acted as if she was already healed. She didn't lie in bed during the day. She got out of bed, bathed, and dressed each morning, despite persisting symptoms of cancer. Although she sometimes cried privately, she decided not to spend much time focused on herself. She felt better when she found ways to minister to others.

Dodie wasn't in denial about what her doctors had told her or the reality of her symptoms. She'd been a registered nurse and one of her sons, a medical doctor, was in the midst of internship that year. She heard him crying outside her hospital room when he first heard about her diagnosis. She *clearly* understood the seriousness of her medical condition, but she refused to let that knowledge dominate her life.

She never did begin chemotherapy (although she recommends that other people do so, if that is recommended by their medical team, because it can be beneficial).

In the early 1980s, God healed Dodie. She felt like David, who wrote: "O Lord my God, I cried to you for help, and you restored my health. You brought me up from the grave, O Lord. You kept me from falling into the pit of death" (Psalm 30:2–3, NLT).

After her requested thirty years of further life had passed, she prayed for many more. Now in her eighties, with nineteen grandchildren, she prays for the healing of countless others.

She followed through on her Psalm 118:17 resolve to recount the deeds of the Lord. She wrote a book called *Healed of Cancer* (which includes letters written by some of her doctors, discussing her diagnosis, prognosis, and full recovery).[18]

Promises, Precedents, Premises, and Prescriptions

When we pray, we can generally remind God of what He said about the nature of His own Word: "… my word… goes out from my mouth; it will not return to me empty, but will accomplish what I desire…" (Isaiah 55:11, NIV) and "… I [God] am watching to see that my word is fulfilled" (Jeremiah 1:12, NIV).

God's words "return" to Him when we include verses in our prayers.

A distinction must be made between promises, precedents, premises, and prescriptions in God's Word. Not every sentence or story in the Bible creates a promise.

Take, for example, the King Hezekiah story. He asked God to give him fifteen more years. God graciously granted that request. Does that story mean that God has automatically promised to do this for all of us? I don't think so. But King Hezekiah's story sets a precedent. The many stories of Jesus healing people also set precedents.

Other verses can be construed as promises. The sentence in 1 Peter 2:24, which states that the wounds of Jesus have healed us, contains a promise.

Some verses are simply premises (general statements or broad propositions), such as the verse we discussed several chapters ago about people usually living until seventy or eighty.

Other verses contain prescriptions. Just as we usually take prescribed medicine, we should diligently do the things that God has prescribed (such as treating our bodies as His temple, getting to know His Word, praying, etc.).

Promises are more powerful than precedents or premises. We can confidently pray: You *promised* in Your Word, in 1 Peter 2:24, that by the wounds of Jesus we *have been* (*are being* and *will be*) healed.

Precedents have a lesser measure of power. I used to plead legal precedents when I presented cases before judges. No judge was bound to follow the precedents I quoted. They could make factual distinctions between the precedents pleaded and the case at hand. But they might be persuaded to follow a particular precedent. They exercised their power as they saw fit.

With my legal background, it's second nature for me to plead biblical precedents in my prayers and then let God decide what He will do. I'm aware that, like human judges, He's not bound to replicate specific precedents.

If we're mentioning the King Hezekiah precedent in our prayers, we can say: God, by Your grace, you gave King Hezekiah additional years after he asked You for them. You did it for him. Can You please do the same thing for me? God also healed David. We can similarly plead with God: You did it for David; please do it for me. Although those precedents do not bind God, perhaps He can be persuaded to follow them. God is the one who supplied us with the precedents.

When we pray about prescriptions, we can ask for God's help in obeying what He has instructed us to do regarding health and healing and other aspects of our lives.

As you encounter hundreds of verses in this book, consider whether they are promises, precedents, premises, or prescriptions. All four kinds of verses have value.

Knowing and Applying the *Whole* Word

It's important to know God's *whole* Word on any topic (as best we can). *Tota Scriptura*. In some ways, the Bible can be compared to a contract. You can't read just *one* sentence, or *one* paragraph, in the Bible *or* in a contract, and think you fully understand what it's saying. It's necessary to read *every*thing a document says on a particular topic to put individual sentences into proper perspective.

While practicing as a lawyer over a few decades, I did a lot of work for insurance clients. I became familiar with a wide range of insurance contracts. A person could buy an "All Risks" policy for their home, which usually contained a lead sentence to this effect: "This policy covers your home against all risks." A person might read that one simple sentence and believe (with a sigh of relief!) that there was no need to read more pages of legal mumbo-jumbo. Wasn't the meaning of the sentence clear and obvious?

Many did not realize the true extent of the insurance coverage on their home until they made a claim for a loss and later received a denial of coverage. The insurer would usually quote sections of the legal mumbo-jumbo that the policyholder had blithely ignored. The Definitions, Limitations, and Exclusions sections of a policy can limit the scope of coverage. Only by reading *all* of those sections can one really understand the extent of actual insurance coverage. A plain sentence ("This policy covers your home against all risks") has to be read in conjunction with the rest of the policy to determine the true meaning and intent of the sentence and the overall policy.

Similarly, the meaning of one sentence in the Bible can only be *fully* understood if one reads the entire document (the whole Bible). Take, for example, the sentence found in 1 Peter 2:24b: "By his [Jesus'] wounds you have been healed." That sentence seems straightforward.

Why not just memorize that verse? Why am I bothering to write a whole book about healing instead of just quoting that one verse? Doesn't that verse say it all? It says a lot, but not everything God has to say on the subject.

That verse mentions nothing about the role of faith in healing, or a person's own responsibility for wise stewardship of their health. We will see that there are hundreds of verses in the Bible that mention such additional dimensions to the subject of healing.

A person can quote that one verse (Peter 2:24), but it will not likely be of much effect if, for example, they are consciously disobeying God, believing that God doesn't heal in this present day, or actively sabotaging their own health.

Let's know God's whole Word and live by it. The better we know it, regarding healing and beyond, the more effectively we can utilize this key point of access to God's healing power. Do not ignore His Word. Do not dismiss it or underestimate it. Choose to believe it, even when it seems fantastical to you. Being well versed will bless you.

Deuteronomy 32:47 proclaims: "For it [God's Word] is no empty word for you, but your very life, and by this word you shall live long..."

10

CHOOSE FAITH

Perhaps you prayed in faith for the healing of a loved one and they died. As we explore the topic of faith, I assure you that I am *not* going to simplistically (or judgmentally) say: "You (or they) must not have had enough faith." Such an attitude would be utterly lacking in understanding and compassion.

Faith is only *one* point of access to God's power to heal. I wouldn't need to write a book of this length if healing relied exclusively on faith. Further, all the faith in the world isn't enough to stop any one of us from eventually dying. Faith isn't a magic elixir that can automatically prevent death the way a medicinal antidote can stop snake poison from killing us.

Faith resides in the deep core of Christian living. Faith doesn't always result in things working out exactly the way we want them to—yet the Bible tells us to choose faith. Even if you think faith has failed you in the past, I invite you to consider it afresh. I promise to later address, from various angles, the disappointment you might bear as a result of seemingly negative faith experiences. Put your hand in His hand as you move through this chapter.

Jesus revealed the potential power of faith on many occasions. Consider, for example, this astounding statement Jesus made: "...

Whatever you ask in prayer, you will receive, if you have faith" (Matthew 21:22).

Jesus further said:

> *... Have faith in God. Truly, I say to you, whoever says to this mountain, "Be taken up and thrown into the sea," and does not doubt in his heart, but believes that what he says will come to pass, it will be done for him. Therefore I tell you, whatever you ask in prayer, believe that you have received it, and it will be yours.*
>
> Mark 11:22–24

The apostle Paul declared:

> *Now faith is the assurance of things hoped for, the conviction of things not seen... And without faith it is impossible to please him [God], for whoever would draw near to God must believe that he exists and that he rewards those who seek him.*
>
> Hebrews 11:1, 6

The KJV refers to faith being the "substance" of what we hope for (v. 1). Faith does indeed have substance and weight. It's real, even though we cannot see it. We can apply faith to every aspect of our Christian lives, including our quest for healing.

Paul wrote: "... we walk by faith, not by sight" (2 Corinthians 5:7). Faith transcends sight. We can possess a spiritual form of sight that's superior to our natural sight. We can imagine ourselves to be healthy again while symptoms of sickness persist.

The four gospels contain so many stories about the role of faith in various healings that we cannot consider them all. We have space to look at just some of them.

Earlier, we discussed a story about a centurion who asked Jesus to heal his servant. Jesus "marvelled" at his faith and said: "'Truly, I tell you, with no one in Israel have I found such faith... And to the centurion Jesus said, 'Go; let it be done for you as you have believed.' And the servant was healed at that very moment" (Matthew 8:10b, 13).

Matthew 9:20–22 reports another story of faith:

And behold, a woman who had suffered from a discharge of blood
for twelve years came up behind him [Jesus] and touched the fringe
of his garment, for she said to herself, "If I only touch his garment,
I will be made well." Jesus turned, and seeing her he said, "Take
heart, daughter; your faith has made you well." And instantly the
woman was made well.

That story is also told in Mark 5:24–34, with a few added details. We learn that the suffering woman had sought help from many doctors. She had spent everything she had on medical care, but to no avail. The more she spent, the worse her condition got. She then decided to place her faith in Jesus. She dared to touch His robe, even though she would have been considered unclean in her state of bleeding (see Leviticus 15:25–27). Jesus rewarded her audacious faith by healing her.

This woman wasn't the only one who touched the garment of Jesus, believing that even that level of encounter was enough to receive healing. Mark 6:56 records: "And wherever he [Jesus] came, in villages, cities, or countryside, they [the crowds] laid the sick in the marketplaces and implored him [Jesus] that they might touch even the fringe of his garment. And as many as touched it were made well." Simply reaching out to touch the clothing of Jesus expressed enough faith for healing to follow.

Others expressed their faith by crying aloud. Matthew 9:27–30 describes two blind men who called out to Jesus for mercy. Jesus asked them this question: "Do you believe that I am able to do this?" (v. 28). When the blind men affirmed their faith in His ability, He touched their eyes and said: "According to your faith be it done to you" (v. 29).

When Jesus healed another blind man, Bartimaeus, He told him: "... Go your way; your faith has made you well" (Mark 10:52). I find the story of Bartimaeus particularly interesting. Before healing him,

Jesus had asked Bartimaeus what he wanted Jesus to do for him (v. 51). Bartimaeus, a roadside beggar, could have asked Jesus for anything, large or small. He could have asked for water to slake his thirst or for money to buy bread. He could have asked Jesus to guide him across the road or for a cloak to keep warm at night. He could have, more daringly, asked for a place to stay. Bartimaeus didn't ask for something small. He asked for something seemingly impossible: to receive his sight again (v. 51). Bartimaeus stretched his faith in Jesus to the max, and Jesus honoured that faith.

Matthew 17:14–18 tells the story of a father who asked Jesus to heal his son. The son suffered greatly from severe seizures, which sometimes caused him to fall into fire or water. The father had previously gone to the disciples of Jesus, but they weren't able to heal his son. Jesus rebuked a spirit in the boy and he was healed. The disciples asked Jesus why they hadn't been able to cast out the spirit and heal the boy. Jesus responded: "… Because of your little faith. For truly, I say to you, if you have faith like a grain of mustard seed… nothing will be impossible for you" (Matthew 17:20–21).

Mark 9 records the story of another father who brought his son to Jesus. The son was epileptic, mute, and deaf. Before healing the boy, Jesus said: "All things are possible for one who believes" (Mark 9:23b). The father honestly responded: "I believe; help my unbelief" (v. 24). None of us has perfect faith. Thankfully, healing doesn't require super faith. We only need faith the size of a mustard seed (which is a very small seed, about the size of the period at the end of this sentence).

Martha, one of three siblings from Bethany who knew Jesus well, expressed radical faith. In John 11:1, we learn that Martha's brother, Lazarus, became sick. Martha and her sister sent word about his illness to Jesus. We know from John 11:5 that "Jesus loved Martha and her sister and Lazarus." Yet surprisingly, Jesus stayed on in another town for a while. Jesus didn't arrive in Bethany until after Lazarus, who had died, had been buried in a tomb for four days.

When He finally showed up in Bethany, Martha hurried to meet Jesus and said to Him: "Lord, if you had been here, my brother would not have died. But even now I know that whatever you ask from God, God will give you" (John 11:21–22). She was fully convinced that Jesus could have healed Lazarus. Even though Lazarus had died, she believed that Jesus could still ask God for a miracle. She had that much faith. You know the end of the story. Jesus raised Lazarus from the dead.

In the stories mentioned so far, faith was either demonstrated by *coming* to Jesus to seek healing, *touching* Him, and/or *verbal* confession that He could heal. On other occasions, people were told to do something else to demonstrate faith. Luke 17:11–14, for example, records:

> *On the way to Jerusalem he [Jesus] was passing along between Samaria and Galilee. And as he entered a village, he was met by ten lepers, who stood at a distance and lifted up their voices, saying, "Jesus, Master, have mercy on us." When he saw them he said to them, "Go and show yourselves to the priests." And as they went they were cleansed.*

The ten men had to leave Jesus and present themselves to their priests, demonstrating their faith by active obedience.

While praying for healing, have you sensed God telling you to do something beyond simply coming to Him in faith or verbally expressing your faith? Do you sense, for example, that you should confess a sin (or two)? Do you know in your gut that you have to make some matter right? Are you being nudged to change some aspect of your lifestyle? We must pay attention to those inner promptings. Perhaps God won't heal your cough until you give up smoking. Perhaps He won't heal your headaches until you forgive someone. Ask Him what He wants you to do and then do it with faith.

Faith Comes from Hearing (Reading) the Bible

Do you struggle to have faith that God can/will heal you or your loved one? We learned earlier that the way to generate faith is by hearing (or reading or recalling) His Word: "So faith comes from hearing, and hearing through the word of Christ" (Romans 10:17). That's why this book is full of Bible verses, references, and stories. I hope that the biblical content you've already encountered has generated faith in you.

Dr. A. B. Simpson, a nineteenth-century pastor and the founder of the Christian and Missionary Alliance, wrote that God's Word, as it pertains to healing, is foundational to true faith for healing. He sent those who inquired about healing to their homes to read God's Word for themselves. He taught that a person ought to be persuaded about what the Bible says about healing before seeking prayer for healing.[19] There is some merit to his stance, although it would not be wrong to pray for the healing of a person who has no knowledge of the Bible.

Maturing in Faith

Faith need not be complicated. Jesus told us that we must become like children if we want to enter His kingdom. I've told you about the disease that afflicted me at the age of nine and about my uncle and my pastor coming to the hospital to pray over me. I responded inwardly to their faith with my own small faith. Now when I imagine coming to God with childlike faith, I recall sitting in my hospital room as a weak little girl. I can still vividly picture that room—where my bed and night table were, the colour of the privacy curtain, the shape of the visitor's chair, where the door was, and much more.

A little seed of faith was planted in some dark soil that day, *deep* in the soil, far from sunlight. But something new definitely pulsed in that gloomy soil. As days passed, I could feel the seed of faith growing little by little. Still surrounded by darkness, it had *life* in it. Over time, the sprouting seed emerged into the light. It blossomed into a growing faith. We might start our Christian journey (and perhaps our healing journey) with a tiny seed of childlike faith, but, over the years, it can mature into a bolder, more confident, knowledge-infused faith.

My husband and I watched our son's faith mature while he battled a health issue, off and on, for a decade. In the last year of that decade, he chose to undergo surgery to deal with that issue. I've already told you that, soon after, he required emergency surgery because of an unexpected complication. (Blood clots had perforated his small bowel, causing abdominal infection and septicemia.) He spent forty days in the hospital, then went through further months of recovery, followed by a third surgery that fall.

The next spring, we witnessed him being baptized, thankful that his faith had remained intact, and had even grown, during his long medical ordeal. Before being dunked in the baptismal pool, he told his church about the health journey that had led to the year of three surgeries. After referencing the "raging storm" he endured that year, he said: "I learned early on in life that in storms like that, my faith became the sails I needed to stay afloat until the storm subsides. Even if those sails became weathered and tattered during the storm, a very small amount [of faith] is enough for God to work with, and He would repair those sails without question."

He further shared: "I felt calm, assured, relaxed, and had a peace beyond understanding going into [the initial] surgery. While things were tougher than anyone expected [after the medical emergency], I had in place both a strong circle of support in our church and my family, and a time-tested faith that allowed me to weather the strongest storm I have faced in my entire life. While I became weak and tired, God used whatever faith I could muster to lift me up and carry me through. And He didn't stop there. He rebuilt my faith and carried me further than I ever could have gone on my own. While all I prayed for was healing and recovery, God gave me so much more…"

He shared about his recovery, becoming engaged, and finding the job of his dreams.

He finished on this note: "I have gone from a child—simply praying for things I wanted, going to Sunday school, and making sure I went to heaven when I died—to realizing that without God in my life, without Jesus in my heart, I don't stand a chance. I am nothing without Jesus. No man on earth or effort of my own can compare to who I am in Jesus. I've realized that without Jesus in my life, the storms would surely continue to come, but I would be not only without sails, but without even a vessel to stay afloat in."[20]

My husband and I rejoice that our son's health has been generally good in the decade since the year of triple surgeries. God has blessed our son with a beautiful wife, two awesome children, a home, and a thriving career. But what we rejoice in most of all is seeing him and his wife continue to mature in their Christian faith.

Resisting Fear

The main enemy of faith is fear. Many people fear sickness and injury. Many also fear death. Some people are so afraid of disease, disability, or death that they become hypochondriacs, worried about the most minor of physical symptoms, scared that every abnormality signals an ominous disease. They read Internet articles, imagine worst-case scenarios, and visit their doctors often. Others go to the opposite extreme and procrastinate about getting medical attention. They suspect that something is wrong but avoid getting confirmation. They don't want to face the feared truth.

Some fear disease and death because of their family history. If a person's parent died of a heart attack at sixty years old, then it's only human for them to feel some fear when they approach their sixtieth birthday. If many relatives have died of cancer, a person might understandably be anxious about the possibility of developing cancer. No profit comes from such fears. Choose to resist them.

A synagogue ruler named Jairus fell at the feet of Jesus, imploring Him to heal his child: "… My little daughter is at the point of death. Come and lay your hands on her, so that she may be made well and live" (Mark 5:23). Someone then came to advise Jairus that his daughter had died. We can only imagine how much that shook the faith of Jairus. At that moment, Jesus said to Jairus: "Don't be afraid; just believe" (Mark 5:36, NIV).

Neither your circumstances nor mine can be any worse than what Jairus was facing when Jesus spoke those words. We need to receive those precious words into our own hearts and minds: "Don't be afraid; just believe." I memorized those five words a long time ago. They have brought me colossal comfort in times of medical crisis.

Don't be afraid. Just believe. Have faith in God. Fix your eyes on Jesus. Stop fixating on your symptoms. We don't have to deny our symptoms, but we don't have to ruminate about them, either. In the middle of the night, when fear can attack with special force, we can choose to meditate on the words of God, not the results of a medical test.

I love hearing present-day stories about people who have chosen faith instead of fear. I watched a news program about a Canadian woman who was lost in the Nevada wilderness for seven weeks. She had no food beyond a little bag of trail mix and a few mints. She swallowed snow for hydration. She lost weight and grew weak. She had a Bible with her that she read every day. She decided to pray and have faith that, against all odds, she would physically survive and eventually be rescued. Her doctors later said that her focus on faith and hope significantly contributed to her survival and recovery.

Resisting Doubt

Another enemy of faith is doubt. It's only human to battle *some* doubt, but battle it we must. Some people spend more time doubting the basis for their faith than they do doubting their doubts.

I like what cancer survivor Dodie learned about doubt. After being diagnosed with metastatic cancer, she encountered a lot of doubt. She then felt self-condemnation over all that doubt. Her husband, a pastor, asked her if the doubt was in her heart or her head. She replied that she had *no* doubt in her heart that God could heal her, wanted to heal her, and would heal her. The doubts all resided in her head. Her husband told her to stop condemning herself. Her faith was intact. She just had to deal with the negative thoughts in her head that assailed her faith. She followed his suggestion to replace those thoughts with daily meditation on helpful Bible passages. God fully healed her.

Resisting Unbelief

A third enemy of faith is unbelief. The New Testament plainly records the great emphasis that Jesus placed on healing the sick. After Jesus ascended, the disciples and apostles of the early church continued to pray for healing. In the first four centuries of the church, most Christ followers prayed for the sick.

Then, for about sixteen centuries, the practice of praying for healing was either neglected or challenged by Catholics and Protestants. Many theologians posited that God's healing power only came down to earth through believers during the days of Jesus, His disciples, and the original apostles of the church. Access to God's healing power through faith and prayer supposedly ceased after that era.

Over a century ago, a revival in believing for healing began, spreading like wildfire in certain denominations. Sparks flew into others. This coincided with a renewed interest in the Spirit and the empowerment that He can give. I encourage you to find a church community that *believes* and teaches God still heals today.

Getting Fresh Perspective on Past Negative Outcomes

I've known people who have died while believing God was going to heal them. Some were still in mid-life or even younger. Perhaps you've encountered similar situations. While I don't pretend to know all of the answers to the questions that arise from such situations, I can hopefully offer a few helpful insights.

It's important to gain some perspective on those seemingly harsh outcomes. We must not let what has happened to others in the past undermine our faith in the present. Just as we don't lose faith in God's promise of salvation because not everyone on earth accepts it, we shouldn't lose our faith in God's healing power just because not everyone on earth gets healed.

Some people abandon their faith after the death of a loved one they prayed for. Charles Darwin (of evolution theory fame) gradually lost his Christian faith. One of the most serious challenges to his faith occurred when God didn't heal his ten-year-old daughter, Annie, from tuberculosis, but instead allowed her to die. Darwin kicked God out of his perception of the universe. While we can empathize with his pain, we don't have to follow his example.

We can gain preliminary perspective on perplexing deaths by examining Hebrews 11, which presents a great list of biblical faith heroes. The apostle Paul wrote that all of them received what they had believed for, but only some received what they believed for in *this* life, while others had to wait until they crossed over into their *eternal* life. Why? I don't know. Paul doesn't explain it. I trust that mysteries such as this will be solved when we meet God face to face.

Hebrews 11 has the power to dispel a lot of confusion, pain, disappointment, and doubt. It can help us believe that those who died while waiting for their healing are now forever free of sickness and pain in heaven.

Should the fact that *some* have to wait until heaven to receive the reward for their faith deter us from having faith for healing in the here-and-now? I don't think so. Hebrews 11 reports that many of the great biblical heroes of faith did receive what they had believed for in *this* life (as have many ordinary people since then). I encourage you to read Hebrews 11 at your leisure. It's not specifically about faith for healing, but it is about faith.

God gets to decide who gets healed in *this* life and who must wait for their restored body in heaven. Don't get stuck on that. Just trust that, one way or another, at one time or another, you or your Christian loved one *will* be healed. Your faith will not be fruitless. I choose to pray in faith for healing this side of glory. What's the downside? God will honour my faith. He will honour yours too. Sooner or later. Here or there.

A friend named Mary received a breast cancer diagnosis. God healed her. Her circle of loved ones rejoiced. But then, about five years later, the cancer returned. Many (including me) joined her in praying for encore healing over the next three years.

God made it clear to Mary about a week before she died that her time had come. She was so sure that He had spoken to her that she sat up in her hospital bed and wrote a letter to be read at her funeral. The gist of her letter, and her subsequent conversations with loved ones that week, proclaimed that our faith-filled prayers for healing are *never in vain*. She thanked God for healing her after her first fight with breast cancer. She thanked Him for sustaining her life for eight years after her initial diagnosis. She thanked Him for many medical miracles, large and small, during those years. She looked forward to her perfect restoration in the life to come. She was at peace that her prayers to be delivered from disease and pain would not be answered until her life in eternity.

I did a lot of thinking after her funeral. What Mary had written made me wonder why we draw an arbitrary line between the life we're granted in this world and the life we're promised in the next. Our lives as Christian believers will be continuous. Our spirits will live on without a pause. We eventually get to exchange our tired, worn-out, old bodies for resurrected bodies that will be indestructible and incorruptible. That sounds like a good deal to me. Why insist on drawing a dark, solid line between one life and the next, as if our next life will be lesser? Why draw any line at all? We can enjoy this life for as long as we have breath, but shouldn't we be joyfully anticipating our seamless transition into our much better life in heaven?

Those thoughts returned one day, years later. While earnestly praying for another woman (much older than Mary) to be healed of her advanced cancer, the Spirit nudged me to pray for her to rise up. Jesus had told sick people to rise up. I repeated those words over and over as I prayed from a distance for the bedridden woman, believing her moment of healing had come.

Later that day, I heard the news that this lovely woman had died during the hour I had been praying. I was momentarily stunned by the news. I asked God: "Why did You tell me to pray for this woman to rise up when You knew You were going to take her this morning? Why? Did I not hear You correctly? Did You not hear me? Was I praying amiss? Why? Why? Why?"

As I poured out my sadness and confusion to God, I felt Him impress these words deep within: "She did rise up, Karen. She did not rise up out of her bed of sickness to you. She rose up to Me. And all is now well." God affirmed what He had taught me through Mary's letter: Our prayers for healing are *never* in vain, even when we don't get the earth-centric outcome we want.

Psalm 73:26 assures us: "My flesh and my heart may fail, but God is the strength of my heart and my portion *forever*." Our faith for healing has to ultimately embrace the *forever* dimension of our journey with God.

We must accept a certain level of mystery in all of this. We'll drive ourselves crazy if we try to figure everything out. We're told in 1 Corinthians 13:12–13: "… now we see in a mirror dimly, but then face to face. Now I know in part; then I shall know fully, even as I have been fully known. So now faith, hope, and love abide…"

We can still seek that *partial* knowledge. God and His ways are not 100 percent mysterious. We can know Him and understand His ways to *some* extent.

We don't know anyone perfectly and completely. I've been married for thirty-five years, and I still don't fully understand my husband. I don't know every detail about his life. I cannot always predict what he will think, say, or do. Yet I still keep trying to know him and understand him. He's not entirely mysterious. Similarly, I can seek to know God and His ways as well as I can.

We can still choose to pray for healing and to believe for healing (with faith, hope, and love), even if we don't completely understand all that God's Word says about healing, or why events unfold as they do, in our lives or in the lives around us.

Let's now examine one further reason that we shouldn't let the deaths of other Christians steal our present faith for healing: We don't usually know the whole story about their spiritual journey, including what they were praying for, from start to finish.

I knew a woman who was diagnosed in her mid-forties with aggressive ovarian cancer. She was initially given only a few weeks to live. Family members and close friends were summoned to her bedside to say goodbye. Some of us didn't say goodbye. Instead, we prayed out loud for her healing, after asking her permission to do so.

This dear woman was miraculously healed and lived for another few years cancer-free. During that time, she gave her testimony in her church. She was shocked and disheartened by the people who later approached her and said hurtful words to this effect: "Who do you think you are? Do you think you're better than brother so-and-so who died of such-and-such, or sister so-and-so who died last year? Why would God heal you and not them? Are you even sure you have been healed?"

When cancer struck again in her late forties, she initially asked family and friends to pray for her healing. Then one day, she told me that she was tired of her pain, tired of chemotherapy, tired of how other Christians challenged her previous healing, and just wanted to "go home" to be with her Lord. Her husband had already picked out his next wife and had told her about his choice. That dispiriting conversation led to her firm decision that she would rather die than carry on. She thanked me for all previous prayers, but said it was her resolute wish that my healing prayers stop then and there. She was fervently asking God to take her to her heavenly home.

Not surprisingly, she died soon after. Many in her church asked why God didn't heal her again. They didn't know about her change of heart. Her death made a lot more sense once they understood. Not everyone got to hear about her desire to "go home." Perhaps to this day some wonder why she wasn't healed a second time.

I've known others who have also changed their minds about seeking healing. Sometimes I'm close enough to hear about it. Other times, I'm praying from a distance and don't know the vicissitudes of the person's own faith, mindset, and desire. Only God truly knows the secrets of the heart.

Let's have faith for healing without being distracted by what has happened to others in the past. One day, we'll better understand what happened to them. One day, we'll hear their whole stories. For now, let's keep our faith focused on the healing matter at hand.

If you insist on thinking about the stories of others, why not think instead about those who did receive healing? For those who don't know anyone who has been healed, I will continue to share positive-outcome stories to offset the seemingly negative outcomes you might have experienced.

Relying on the Faith of Others

When we pray for healing, there might be times when we need to rely on the faith of others. Perhaps even now you're too sick, too tired, or in too much pain to muster up much faith of your own. Perhaps you're groggy with medication. Maybe you struggle with discouragement.

James 5:14–16 refers to the faith of a *community* of believers. The elders of the church are instructed to pray for the sick. We learn that the faith-filled prayers of those in right standing with God are powerful and effective when seeking healing for the sick.

One benefit of being in a church community is that the whole burden of having faith for healing is not up to us alone. Others can bring *their* faith to bear. I freshly encourage you to attend a church where most people believe in God's healing power.

Imparting Faith to Others

While still a young pastor in his twenties, A. B. Simpson developed serious heart trouble. He barely had the strength to speak at three services a week—two on Sunday and another one mid-week. He prayed in faith for healing for more than a decade.

Despite ongoing weakness and fatigue, Simpson maintained his belief that healing was a part of the gospel and an aspect of the redemption offered by Christ. After *years* of praying, God healed him at the age of thirty-seven. Over the next three years, he preached over a thousand sermons, sometimes speaking at twenty services per week. His healing increased his strength, but it also increased his faith and his capacity to pray for the healing of others.[21]

Oral Roberts was healed of both tuberculosis and stuttering at the age of seventeen, after his brother took him to a meeting where an evangelist was praying for the sick. Roberts went on to develop a significant healing ministry of his own over later decades, reaching millions through radio, television, books, and services.[22]

Once we have exercised faith for a healing that comes to us, our faith can be replicated. We can passionately (and compassionately) support others in their healing journeys. Through prayer, encouragement, teaching, and testimony, we can impart our faith to others.

Seeing Ourselves Well

When a health crisis strikes, I've learned not to waste valuable time and energy asking "why" (Why this? Why me? Why now?). What's the point? Why not choose to skip those questions and instead focus on faith?

With faith, we can imagine ourselves (or a loved one) looking well again. Though pale, tired, and bedridden, we can imagine playing our favourite sport again, full of strength and energy. We can visualize a future that's different from the present (without denying what's currently happening).

The woman who had been bleeding for twelve years did just that as she crawled forward to touch the robe of Jesus, stating that she would be well if she touched Him. She could imagine herself being well again, even though she'd been sick for so long. She was fully aware of her condition, but she had faith that her condition could change.

We don't need to deny that our sickness exists. We just need to deny its ongoing right to exist in our bodies. We can refuse to put out the welcome mat that invites sickness to stay. We can instead choose to exercise faith that He will heal us one day.

11

PRAY

At the Atlanta airport, I received news via email that my dear friend and prayer partner, Shirley, had suffered a cardiac event at the age of sixty-eight. Shirley had gone to the hospital, complaining of severe chest pain. The emergency doctor determined that she had suffered a heart attack.

Because of that email, I prayed for Shirley while waiting to board my flight. Just after boarding, a baggage cart driver ran recklessly into one of the plane's wings, damaging and disabling it. All passengers had to deplane and wait for another flight. I had five further hours to pray that afternoon in the airport.

When I visited Shirley the next day in the cardiac ICU, she told me she needed triple bypass surgery. The state of her body presented a few unusual complications that would make that imminent surgery even riskier than usual.

I prayed with her in person during that first visit. It felt a little strange, praying with her in that hospital room after many years of praying with her in the comfort of her living room. After I left, I privately pled with God yet again to spare her life. I couldn't imagine losing such a special friend.

The cardiac surgery took hours. Post-surgery, Shirley developed pericarditis (inflammation around the heart) that eventually required a few more hospitalizations. I visited her further times in the hospital and in her home. She looked and sounded frail. Health and strength can dissipate so quickly.

It took months for the stubborn inflammation around her heart to subside. During that time, Shirley suffered significant pain, prolonged immobility, circulatory problems, a swollen leg, shortness of breath, fluid build-up pressing against her lungs, and weight loss. At one point, she told me she weighed less than one hundred pounds.

As prayer partners, we'd prayed so often in the past for healing—sometimes for ourselves, and other times for family members. During her heart crisis and recovery, when I prayed for her alone at home, I could almost hear her voice. I could imagine what *she* would pray. I knew the favourite verses we usually recited in our joint prayers and the customary words we spoke as we asked God for healing. Even when she couldn't be with me, I knew she'd agree with the way I was praying for her.

She'd always been such a faithful prayer warrior, touching my life with her prayers. She'd prayed for my husband, my father, and my son during many of the hospitalizations I've described in this book, and for many other family members when they had health problems. We had, of course, also prayed together for her family. Together we had seen some glorious answers to prayer.

Shirley had led church prayer groups and taught classes on prayer. She'd prayed for our church, its congregants, and our nation. It's rare to find someone with such a heart for prayer. Surely God could still use her in such vital ministry.

I prayed often for her. Sometimes I phoned her so she could hear me praying out loud. Of course, many others also prayed. No doubt some prayed with even greater frequency and fervency. Shirley prayed too. God heard all of us. Power was released for a great measure of healing.

I write this chapter with passion. I have experienced firsthand the power of prevailing prayer on occasions too numerous to count. Prayer has been integral to every personal story I'm sharing with you.

Prayer has played a major part in the stories about other people that you will discover in this book. Dodie, for example, relentlessly prayed during her cancer battle. She prayed alone in the middle of the night and throughout each day. She also prayed with her husband, family, and many other people.

Why doesn't everyone pray for healing? The number of Christians I meet who *don't* pray for healing, and who are not receptive to anyone else praying with them, astounds me. Perhaps their theology resists it. Perhaps they've accepted their injury or illness as their lot in life. I don't want to sound critical. I understand how easy it is to feel tired, defeated, or convinced that there's no point in praying. I hope, in this chapter, to encourage every reader to pray, to allow yourself to be prayed for by others, and to step out to pray for those in need.

Prayer is one of the most important points of access to God's mighty healing power. Jesus promised: "And whatever you ask in prayer, you will receive, if you have faith" (Matthew 21:22). Enormous power can be released when a faith-filled person prays with boldness and expectancy.

The story of King Hezekiah demonstrates the power of prayer. After King Hezekiah prayed, asking God to heal him, God instructed the prophet Isaiah, who was leaving the King's palace: "Turn back [Isaiah], and say to Hezekiah the leader of my people... I [the Lord] have heard your prayer; I have seen your tears. Behold, I will heal you" (2 Kings 20:5a).

King David affirmed the effectiveness of praying for healing: "O Lord my God, I cried to you for help, and you have healed me" (Psalm 30:2).

Praying to the Father in the Name of Jesus

Christians are instructed to pray to Father God in the name of Jesus (see, for example, John 14:13). Through Christ, we have privileged access to the Father. To know that we are praying to our heavenly *Father*, not to some cold and impersonal deity, comforts me. We can speak to God the same way we can speak to our human father. (If you haven't had a loving father, try to imagine what such a father might be like.)

Timothy Keller wrote in his book, *Prayer*, that praying in the name of Jesus is an abbreviated way of pleading His divine status and what He has done for us.[23]

At times, we can directly address Jesus, or the Spirit, in our prayers. J. I. Packer wrote that normally we pray to the Father, through the Son, enabled by the Spirit. But Packer believes that we can pray directly to Jesus or the Spirit, when appropriate.[24] For example, the New Testament tells us that many people asked Jesus for healing, providing precedent for us to ask Him directly too.

Prayer Forms

The Lord's Prayer, found in Matthew 6, provides a useful template for prayer. Words taken straight out of the Lord's Prayer contain peerless potency. We can pray, for example, these four words found in Matthew 6:13: "… deliver us from evil." If you think cancer is evil, then ask God to deliver you from it. Something is either good or evil. I cannot imagine any argument in support of cancer being good.

We can pray in a less-structured way. Honest and sincere words of our own can flow from our heart. Our words aren't limited by any formula. Although I include sample prayers for healing at the end of this book, I don't pretend to know any magic or mandatory words.

You can pray in accordance with the Christian faith tradition with which you're most comfortable. You might have grown up with a lot of liturgy. It's fine to quote familiar words that you have recited in church over and over. Or you might have grown up in an atmosphere of freestyle prayer. That's fine too. God cares about the substance of our prayers, not fancy wording. We don't have to strain to sound eloquent, saintly, or fresh out of seminary. We can be ourselves in the presence of God.

Scripture-Based Prayer

I encourage you to quote scripture in your prayers, using God's own words to state your case for healing. God's words pack a much greater punch than our own. If you pray using your own words, frame your prayers based on what you know to be true about God and His ways.

In his excellent book, *Prayer*, Timothy Keller believes our prayers should be our response to the biblically revealed knowledge we have of God. Our prayer impact is affected by the amount of knowledge we have and how accurate it is. Keller cautions that prayers not grounded in God's Word might be based on our notions of who we would like God to be, instead of who He actually is.[25] (Keller, by the way, battled thyroid cancer. The last I heard, he is cancer-free.)

The more often we read the whole Bible right through, the more we'll learn about God. We'll encounter the prayers of others and can examine how they approached God. We can learn from Abraham, Moses, Job, David, and Paul, among many others. The Bible records what they prayed about and the manner in which they conversed with God.

David, for example, demonstrated that we can incorporate some lament into our prayers, thereby releasing some of our pain. David often lamented (see, for example, his prayers in Psalm 22 and 88). David moaned about his soul being discouraged and downcast. He complained about his emotional pit. At times, David sounds hopeless, maybe even depressed. Telling God about our authentic feelings *is* allowed. But take note that David often ended a psalm by saying that he would *yet* find his hope in God, that he would *yet* have reason to praise Him. David avoided getting stuck in anger, sadness, fear, or despair. So go ahead and pray some words of lamentation. Use some of David's words if they resonate with you. If your pain is raw, or your suffering is suffocating, tell God about it, but try to end such lament on a positive note.

The ACTS Model of Prayer

I often give my prayers balanced structure by following the ACTS acronym. (I don't know whom to credit for this model of prayer that I was introduced to years ago.)

A stands for **adoration**. Let us adore God in prayer, acknowledging the nature of the person to whom we are speaking. Let's worship Him as the God of unlimited power, our Creator and sustainer, ruler of the whole universe, Lord of lords, and King of kings. Let's adore His character attributes, such as His love, compassion, kindness, empathy, mercy, and grace. Let's focus on the *presence* of God, not rushing this stage of prayer. John Calvin called approaching God with awe and reverence his first rule of prayer.[26]

C signifies **confessing** our sins. James 5:14–16 establishes that we should confess our sins when we ask God for healing. We must primarily confess our sins to God but also to others, if appropriate. Unless we are prepared to confess our sins *and* turn away from them, we cannot expect God to answer our prayers for healing. Although, by His grace and mercy, God sometimes heals unrepentant sinners, He has warned us that sin can block our prayers. If you don't know God, or if you've lived a sin-filled life in disregard of Him, God may or may not bend His ear to your prayers. I encourage you to get right with God if you want Him to hear your petition for healing. Your spiritual healing is most important and most urgent. Acquiring spiritual health may have to precede the restoration of your physical health.

T represents **thanksgiving**, an important but often neglected aspect of prayer (and our Christian walk in general). We will commit a whole chapter to it.

S stands for **supplication**. As suppliants, we petition God, making our requests and needs known, while crying out for His help. We can make specific supplication regarding every troublesome sign and symptom of our medical condition (such as fever, inflammation, infection, or pain). No detail is too small. We can also ask God to shine His light (His revelation) on our medical condition so that our doctor(s) can make the right diagnosis and provide the best treatment. We can ask Him to grant the doctor(s) knowledge, insight, wisdom, good judgment, skill, and diligence.

Supplication doesn't require grovelling. The effectiveness of our supplications will *not* depend on the length of time we pray or on weeping and wailing. Jesus said in Matthew 7:7 to simply ask and we will receive. Jesus did not say that we should grovel or beg.

This chapter will mostly address supplication, but let us remember that supplication can be accompanied by adoration, confession, and thanksgiving. This balanced structure in prayer is for our own good. If our entire prayer consists of supplication, we will remind ourselves of our needs, of what is lacking, of what is wrong in our lives. If all we do is list our problems, we can leave a time of prayer feeling heavy, weary, and anxious, maybe even overwhelmed. Confession lightens our spiritual load. Adoration and thanksgiving turn our attention to what is positive about God and His dealings with us. If we add adoration, confession, and thanksgiving into the mix, we can often leave our prayer time feeling refreshed and unburdened.

Praying for Others

We can learn how to intercede (pray) for others. Intercession becomes especially important when the brain of the sick, injured, or medicated person fires on only half of its pistons. Or perhaps the person might be unconscious and cannot pray. Or maybe the ailing person doesn't know how to pray.

Abraham successfully interceded for the healing of King Abimelech and his household (Genesis 20:17). Isaac interceded for his wife, Rebekah, who was childless: "And the Lord granted his prayer, and Rebekah his wife conceived" (Genesis 25:21).

While on this earth, Jesus responded to people who sought healing on behalf of loved ones. For example, someone asked Jesus to heal Peter's mother-in-law, who was sick in bed with a fever (Luke 4:38). We've discussed Jairus coming to Jesus on behalf of his dying young daughter (Mark 5:21–42). Jesus healed their loved ones. We can't approach Jesus as a man on earth anymore, but we can approach Him (and Father God and the Holy Spirit) in prayer.

The apostle John interceded for others. He wrote in his letter to Gaius: "Beloved, I pray that all may go well with you and that you may be in good health, as it goes well with your soul" (3 John 1:2).

I know a woman who was born with good sight but became blind as a young child. Neither she nor her family were believers at that time, but they had a Christian neighbour who prayed for her healing. Later in her childhood, she unexpectedly recovered her sight. This influenced her eventual decision to become a Christian. It may be that her neighbour was the only person who prayed for her.

Another friend of mine lost her eyesight after a stroke. Her medical team didn't expect that she would recover her sight. She prayed, but also asked many others to pray for her. Her doctors were quite amazed when her eyesight was soon restored.

One of my early experiences in intercessory prayer left a deep impression on my spirit, helping me to develop confidence as an intercessor. I wrote earlier about a woman who had advanced ovarian cancer. She was told she had a few weeks to live. Her husband summoned close family members and friends to say goodbye. I became part of a small group that chose to pray in agreement for her healing. She went on to live, medically inexplicably, for another four years. After that experience, I became bolder whenever I prayed for the healing of others.

You might be hesitant to pray for others if you're inexperienced. In Appendices B and D, I provide sample intercessory prayers that allow you to fill in the name of the person you're praying for and details about them. In time, if you pray for others often, you'll become adept at framing effective intercessory prayers in your own words.

We must always pray for others in a loving spirit. Jesus taught that the second greatest commandment in the whole Bible is to love others as we love ourselves (Matthew 22:39). We should do everything, including praying for healing, as an act of love. We must not pray out of arrogance, self-importance, self-righteousness, or pride. If we pray in a loving tone for someone, they may sense God's love. Imagine being a human conduit for the flow of God's superlative, supreme, incomparable love.

If present with the person in need, we can invite them to pray with us (if they are able to). What if we're halfway across the globe? Intercessors don't need to be physically present with the person they're praying for.

When we pray for the healing of others, we should ask God for wisdom and discernment *before* we ask for healing. We don't know every detail about the person we're praying for, no matter how well we think we know them. In a later chapter, we'll talk about common obstacles to healing. Many reasons exist regarding why God doesn't heal some individuals or doesn't heal them right away. We don't always know if one or more obstacles are present in the life of the person we're praying for. We cannot know for certain if God will choose to heal the person we're praying for. God might be more interested, in the short term, in bringing pressure to bear on the ailing person so that they seek to remove whatever obstacles are blocking His healing power in their lives.

If we're aware of some obstacles present in the individual's life, we can pray for specific obstacle removal. We can also pray for their healing. God is full of surprises. I have seen Him heal people: who do not believe in Him; who, even if they do believe in Him, do not believe that God still heals today; or who are deeply mired in sins of various kinds.

If I'm aware of obstacles, I'll ask for healing based on God's love, mercy, and grace, but I won't pray with the same kind of authority I might use in other situations. I wouldn't have the full expectation that God will heal the person whose life displays some serious obstacles that separate them from God's loving desire to heal them.

Because we don't know everything about the person we're praying for, and because God will do what He wants, we must pray for others with humility. Our job is to pray. We don't know how, if, or when God will answer our prayer for healing. The results of our prayers are always up to Him. He knows the person we're praying for inside out. God alone can decide whether any obstacles are serious enough to prevent or delay healing. He can override the obstacles if He wants to.

In Francis MacNutt's books on healing, he talks often about the worldwide renewal of interest in (and passion for) praying for the sick. According to him, prior to the mid-1970s, many of his fellow Catholics didn't feel comfortable about praying for physical healing. This has changed dramatically.[27]

When MacNutt was much younger, he believed one had to be a saint (in the capital "S" sense of the word) to ask God to heal someone. He hadn't been trained in seminary to pray for the sick. Over time, he grew in faith that even he, as an ordinary Christian, could pray for the healing of others. So he stepped out to pray. God taught him through extensive experience that He *does* hear the prayers of ordinary people. MacNutt further learned that praying for others doesn't necessarily signal that we are full of pride in our spiritual prowess.[28] We can pray with an awareness that we are sinners saved by grace, with the focus being on God's healing power, not on our spiritual maturity.

MacNutt has pointed out that we should not assume that we are the right person to pray for *every* sick person we hear about. We shouldn't spread ourselves too thin, draining our energy to the point of depletion. I keep on referring to praying for loved ones because, first and foremost, we should pray for those we truly love. Of course, we can pray for those we know less well, but we should seek God on this. Are we at peace praying for the person in question? Have they asked us to pray? What do we know about their situation? Do we feel faith welling up within? Has God given us particular compassion or empathy for them? Has He nudged us to pray?

We can ask the person *if* they want us to pray for healing. I remind you about the woman who died of ovarian cancer after it recurred.

You might recall that she told me she no longer wanted to be healed but, instead, wanted to "go home" to be with her Lord. There's no point wasting energy praying at odds with what the sick person clearly desires.

To learn more about intercessory prayer, you can read books such as Andrew Murray's *With Christ in the School of Prayer* and Dutch Sheets' *Intercessory Prayer*.

Praying for Ourselves

We can, of course, pray for our own selves. In Appendices B and C, I provide sample prayers you can pray if you're not comfortable framing your own prayer. You can modify these prayers, using your own words and adding specific details about your health condition.

Don't carry around the *burden* of your sickness or injury or disability. By the act of prayer, give your burden to God. In 1 Peter 5:7, we're told to cast all of our cares upon Him, because He cares for us. We can train ourselves to constantly do that. We can cast our infirmity on Him, and also our fear, frustration, confusion, and whatever other thoughts and feelings might be disturbing us during a medical challenge.

At age seventy, my friend and prayer partner, Shirley, had to undergo a series of two angioplasties and stent procedures to deal with three blocked arteries. Going into those procedures, she was considered high-risk (for complications or death) because just a few years earlier, she had undergone triple bypass surgery.

During the first angioplasty and stent procedure, the cardiac surgeon perforated one of Shirley's arteries. Her blood pressure kept dropping as the surgeon tried to patch it. Shirley was conscious enough to hear the surgeon tell his team a few times, "It's dropping." Detecting the urgent tone of his voice, Shirley immediately prayed, thankful she hadn't been fully anaesthetized. Days later, the surgeon told Shirley that he thought he'd almost lost her a few times while trying to patch the perforated artery. He considered the fact that he was able to save her life a "miracle." (Of course, Shirley would say it was *God* who saved her life!)

Many of us prayed for Shirley that morning, but I believe *her* prayers, pleading with God for her own life, mattered most of all. In any situation in which we are conscious, we can and should pray for our own health and healing.

Verbally Declaring God's Healing Power

Proverbs 18:21 advises: "Death and life are in the power of the tongue..." Do we really grasp what this means? In an earlier chapter, we talked about praying scripture out loud. We can also pray our own heart-felt words out loud. Our *spoken* prayers (even if we're the only one in the room) might help us to feel increased faith.

Praying out loud can increase the faith of a sick person who is listening. I remember how I felt, five decades ago, when my uncle and my pastor prayed for me while I lay in a hospital bed. I'm so glad they prayed audibly instead of just quietly in their own hearts. Their spoken words mattered.

This makes me think of a ministry leader I know named Shaila. In 2011, she was hospitalized for a life-threatening illness called cryptococcal meningitis. A spreading ball of fungus had formed near the base of her brain. The doctors told her she would likely be in the hospital for at least eight weeks and might require brain surgery to remove the fungal ball. Many people began praying for her.

On Good Friday, her pastor visited. She'd been in the hospital for about five weeks. He prayed for her. He told her he believed God was going to heal her, even though he hadn't made that kind of statement to others in the past. She admits her own faith for healing wasn't very strong at that time. (She had lost a good friend to cancer the year before.)

Soon after the Easter weekend, one of her doctors reported new MRI results, which indicated all traces of the fungal invasion were gone. Not even a scar remained where the fungal ball had been. The doctor couldn't explain this sudden development. He said it was as if she had never had the fungal mass. He discharged her that very day.

Unity in Prayer: Two or More Praying in Agreement

I've come to understand the exponential power of united prayer. That's why I regularly spend time with a prayer partner. Jesus told His followers:

> *Again, truly I tell you that if two of you on earth agree about any-thing they ask for, it will be done for them by my Father in heaven. For where two or three gather in my name, there am I with them.*
> Matthew 18:19–20, NIV

When Sam was in ICU, I prayed the first night with our adult kids. I also immediately initiated prayer chains, involving further family members and friends. Within twenty-four hours, hundreds were praying in accordance with my specific requests. Texts and emails confirming prayer support inundated my cell phone. Messages filled my answering machine at home. Over the following days, many family members and friends came to pray with us in person at the hospital. I believe that all that prayer mattered.

You might think you have enough faith to pray on your own and never need the help of others, but God has told us we *need* the support of other believers. Individuals do not have anywhere near the same power as united prayers of agreement.

Be careful whom you ask to pray with you, especially if they will pray in your physical presence. Surround yourself with people who will *support* your prayer requests. You want those who will *affirm* your faith for healing and who will pray in true agreement. Airing theological differences about healing can wait for another time.

You can ask for the elders of your church to pray for you or your loved one (as we are instructed to do in James 5:14) if your church believes in God's healing power. Otherwise, you can look for a healing service at some other church, where there is a faith-filled environment and a prayer time.

I'm thankful for websites that facilitate intercessory prayer in cyberspace. One example is caringbridge.org.[29] You can go on that website and set up your own page (for yourself or a loved one). Family and friends can be invited to participate on that page. Regular reports regarding the sick person's progress, along with specific prayer requests, can be posted on the page (which becomes a series of pages). In response, family and friends can post their written prayers and comments of support and encouragement. Hundreds of people can get involved. A caring community can evolve. This process saves the tiring effort of having to phone or email a long list of individuals to update them. I know how exhausting it can be to keep a whole bunch of people in the loop when a loved one is sick or hospitalized for a lengthy period. Having to respond to numerous texts, emails, cards in the mail, and voicemail messages can be overwhelming!

I participated on an interactive digital page while a friend of mine experienced her cancer journey. Daily I observed how much prayer, love, and comfort were generated by her caring community. My friend valued the thousands of posts. Those posts also strengthened her husband and daughter, who faithfully sat by her hospital bed for several months.

Posting medical updates and prayer requests to a defined group of social media friends provides another way to generate united prayer. Not everyone can visit a sick person, but they can send love and prayers across the miles through social media.

Another resource is Stormie Omartian's website, where you can post prayer requests.[30] Many unnamed prayer warriors will pray in agreement with you. I received thousands of intercessory prayers (for myself and loved ones) on that site over a five-year period (which included the weeks when my father, husband, and son were in life-threatening situations in ICU wards). I kept a journal of my requests and the number of people who prayed for each item. I saw blessing and breakthrough in so many areas of our lives, including our health needs.

I recommend that site to anyone going through a medical crisis who urgently (maybe desperately) desires extensive intercessory prayer.

I first posted requests to Stormie's prayer community just before the forty-day hospitalization of our son. I thereafter went on that site at least once a day (sometimes hourly when our son was in critical condition), making one specific request after another. Every time I clicked "send," I felt immense relief that others were going to share my burdens. Sometimes they carried those burdens when I couldn't. People in other time zones would pray while I slept. I would wake up to discover that, overnight, dozens of people had prayed for each request. They also prayed during those moments in the daytime when I felt too discouraged or weary to pray. Imagine the synergistic power of the thousands of intercessory prayers that accumulated over time. We should never underestimate the *exponential* value of *many* people praying.

Scientific Studies on the Effects of Prayer

At least a few hundred scientific/medical studies have established that prayer promotes better health for the person who prays. In addition, more than one hundred controlled studies have been conducted to consider what effect the intercessory prayer of others has on a person's healing. More than half of them present statistical proof that prayer has a significant impact.[31]

Studies exist that cast doubt on the positive effects of prayer. Some of those studies involved people who didn't know they were being prayed for and who may not have prayed for themselves. Not all such studies are linked to Christian prayer, or biblically sound prayer, or prayer based on the belief that God still heals today. When relying on a study (to either "prove" or "disprove" the effects of prayer), it's important to understand the details of the study.

We don't need scientific evidence to motivate our spiritual practices, but I find it interesting that *many* medical studies affirm prayer's positive impact on the healing process.

The Necessity of Prayer

Jesus Himself, the Son of God, prayed to the Father regularly. After Jesus healed a leper: "… even more the report about him [Jesus] went abroad, and great crowds gathered to hear him and to be healed of their infirmities. But he [Jesus] would withdraw to desolate places and pray" (Luke 5:15–16).

Jesus needed time alone with His Father. He was then ready to face the crowds and their needs again. Luke 5:17b talks about how, after Jesus had withdrawn for a while to pray, "the power of the Lord was with him to heal." His power while here on earth appears to have been recharged by His prayer life.

If Jesus needed to pray so that people could be healed, how much more do we? So let's pray, pray, pray. James 4:2b states: "You do not have, because you do not ask." Jesus instructed: "Ask, and it will be given to you…" (Matthew 7:7a).

Letting Go

Prayer for healing should *not* be about performing and achieving, succeeding or failing. The results are always as God decrees. The healing process is up to Him, not us. Every time we pray, we can *let go* (of our burdens, anxieties, and need to control the situation) and *let God* work. God will answer our prayers when, how, and in what measure He chooses. The outcome is in His hands.

I love what Revelation 8:4 says about our prayers: They rise as incense before the throne of God and His angelic host. Can you imagine that? Every good prayer you have ever prayed has risen up to His throne in heaven, as a sweet fragrance that lingers until it has been answered as our wise, loving, gracious, and merciful God wishes.

12

CHOOSE TRUST

Before our son's year of surgeries, our family vacationed in Florida. One day, we all sat on lounge chairs by the pool. While trying to relax, I found myself distracted. Our son hadn't been feeling well that week. I silently prayed for him.

As I prayed, I looked up into the clear blue sky and noticed a small airplane. The plane began to whirl and twirl, writing some white-smoke letters across the skyscape. I watched as the acrobatic plane slowly spelled out "T-R-U-S-T." I cynically wondered what business was about to solicit my trust. The plane left some blue space after the second "T." Then, I saw the letter "J" form. I guessed, immediately, that further plane-scribed letters would spell "J-E-S-U-S."

TRUST JESUS. Written across the sky in bold letters. Those words soothed my heart. In that surreal moment, I knew that our son's health was going to be okay. I sensed that he was going to recover soon (which he did). All I had to do was trust Him (so simple, yet sometimes so difficult).

A few years later, I stood in the hall outside the operating room where our son was undergoing emergency surgery. You might recall that the surgery was urgent because his small bowel had perforated after an earlier surgery, dangerously spilling bacteria into his abdomen and bloodstream.

Just before my son had been wheeled into the operating room, our eyes had briefly locked. The nurse had stopped his gurney beside me long enough for my son to tell my husband and I to stay strong. I hadn't been able to hug him because he was then whisked past me. Instead, I reached for his hand as I tried to keep pace with the moving gurney.

I cannot describe the enormity of my pain as I let go of his hand and watched the gurney disappear into the operating room. I also felt overwhelmed as I thought about the seriousness of the situation. I tried to push worst-case scenarios out of my mind.

After the operating room doors closed, I stood motionless in the hall, my husband beside me, struggling with his own thoughts. It was early evening, and the starkly lit hospital corridor was quiet and empty. With nary a chair in sight, I leaned my upper back against one of the drably painted walls.

As I closed my eyes and tried to pray, an image began forming in my mind. I wasn't summoning the image. It seemed to be summoning me. I could see blue sky, lit up with brilliant summery sunshine. Could this be an image of heaven? Then I saw a small airplane soundlessly writing two mighty words across the sky: TRUST JESUS. I mentally snared those white-smoke words on the backdrop of my closed eyelids. They offered me a precious lifeline.

Somehow, I had known a few years before that the plane-scribed words I'd seen in Florida weren't just meant for that time and place. I had sensed that the words provided a divine instruction for the future, a future in which Jesus would show up with a great display of power. A God who writes visible words up in the sky for His hurting daughter to read is a God willing to engage in further wonder-working ways down here on this earth.

That once-vague future had arrived in the bleak hospital corridor. As my husband and I waited hours for the surgery to end, we knew we had to trust Jesus more than ever. Our son was under anaesthesia, no longer able to place his own conscious trust in God. We would have to trust Jesus on his behalf.

Jesus had known all along that it would be difficult for me to trust Him in those hours. That's probably why He'd arranged, a few years before through some human servant of His, to write a strength-infusing message in the stratosphere. I could, of course, read about trusting God in my Bible any day of the week. In that hallway, I could have taken out my mobile phone and clicked on my digital Bible. But *remembering* the two words so grandly written in giant letters up there in His vast celestial sky reminded me of how powerful, loving, and caring He is. The extraordinary memory granted me enough strength to trust Him at such a critical time. I wouldn't let go of those cloud-white words in my mind. I focused on them with all my being.

Hours passed—hours that would have been unbearably nerve-wracking had I not had those words writ across the blue firmament. Every time fear, panic, or despair threatened to seep into my mind, I chose to block such thoughts and feelings. I chose instead to trust Jesus, one agonizing moment at a time.

Finally, the lead surgeon emerged from the operating room. He approached my husband and I with a poker face. I had no idea what he was going to say. All I could cling to was my resolve to trust Jesus.

The surgeon told us our son had lived through the surgery and would be moved to an ICU recovery room. The surgeon couldn't assure us that all would be well. Some infection had been cleaned out of his abdominal cavity, but a large amount of infection had already poisoned his bloodstream. "Time will tell what will happen" was his ultimate message. It didn't bring comfort. My focus reverted to the two words I had been gifted with, words that *did* bring comfort.

After a while, we were allowed into the recovery room. Our son lay there, still intubated. His arms were strapped tightly to the sides of his bed. He was trying to break his arms free so that he could pull the irritating plastic tube out of his mouth. When he couldn't release his arms, he mouthed some words. It was hard to figure out what he was trying to say with that big tube taking up most of his mouth, and his dry throat unable to produce any audible sound. Finally, I could make out his mimed message: Help me.

Help me, he kept soundlessly pleading. *Trust Jesus*, I kept thinking. That was all I could do, for him and for me. Our son's blood pressure soared. He was frustrated and agitated because we wouldn't release his arms from their constraints or remove the uncomfortable tube from his mouth. I realized, even before the nursing staff told us, that it would be best for our son if we left him for the night. The surgeon had told us that if our son survived, he would be hospitalized for another several weeks. The nurses strongly encouraged my husband and I to go home to get some sleep. I cannot express how tough it was to leave our son's side while his life hung in the balance and while he was still mouthing a plea for help.

As we left the hospital, Sam surmised (based on what the surgeon had told him and on his own doctorly instincts) that there was a fifty-fifty chance we would see our son alive the next morning. Those were heart-strangling words. I wondered if I could keep breathing after I heard them.

My husband and I drove home in the separate cars we had arrived in earlier that day. I prayed all the way home. Three wordscapes battled to take over my mind: the calming image of the words "Trust Jesus" written across my mental sky; the memory of my son mouthing the words, "Help me"; and the image of my husband woodenly stating, "He might die in the night." I couldn't refute the reality of the medical situation, but I *could* choose to keep trusting Jesus. So I did.

It was during that long drive home that I also remembered Psalm 23:4, about God shepherding us through the valley of the *shadow* of death. That fourth wordscape vied for space in my mind. I decided I would not fear a dark shadow.

After the emergency surgery, our son spent a few days in the ICU (with one-on-one nursing care), then several weeks in step-down intensive care (one nurse per two patients). Infection still raged in his abdomen and bloodstream. Our son continued to fight for his life. I continued to focus on trusting Jesus, who remained my security, stability, and sanity.

Psalm 37:5 states: "Commit your way to the Lord; trust in him, and he will act." Proverbs 3:5 advises: "Trust in the Lord with all your heart, and do not lean on your own understanding." So many other verses instruct us to trust God (Father, Son, and Spirit).

Choosing trust was sometimes very tough. In the early weeks, our son kept spiking high fevers. His bed linens became so soaked with the resulting perspiration that they had to be changed several times a day. His heart rate and blood pressure also spiked to alarming levels. (My own blood pressure probably rose whenever I looked at his vital stats on the bedside monitor.) Even when given the maximum dose of narcotic medication, he endured significant pain. He had drainage tubes sticking out of open incisions in his chest.

For days he couldn't eat. When finally allowed to eat, he didn't have an appetite. Eating caused pain. He lost forty pounds, about one quarter of his pre-hospital weight. He had such little padding on his butt that it hurt to sit, even on a soft chair. He looked pale and gaunt. It was hard to trust God in those miserable circumstances.

We place faith in His Word, but *trust* must primarily be in God Himself, in His character, His track record, and His gracious intentions.

When you're suffering, do you find it hard to trust God? To trust that He even exists? That He is all-powerful? That He is loving, kind, compassionate, merciful, and full of grace? That He can heal and wants to heal? Tough circumstances make it tough to trust Him. I know.

One evening about halfway through our son's hospitalization, I briefly left his room in the step-down ICU. When I returned, a windowless metal door had been rolled across the entrance to the step-down ward. Discovering that the door was locked, I sensed that something horrible must be happening on the other side of it. Only two nurses and four patients, including my son, had been behind that locked door moments before. It took all of my effort to focus on trusting God instead of fearing the worst.

When the door finally opened, I was so relieved to find out that our son was okay. The patient in the room beside him, a man named Luigi, was not so fortunate. He had died while I had stepped out of the ward. A priest and weeping family members later gathered around Luigi's bedside, trying to trust God in their much more difficult circumstances.

We must trust Him in the midst of chaos and confusion, even when circumstances deteriorate, even when worst-case scenarios do come to pass. We must trust Him when we cannot control what's happening. We must trust that He remains in ultimate control. We must trust Him even when He doesn't answer our prayers the *way* we want, *when* we want.

Years ago, I memorized this verse, found in Isaiah 26:3–4: "You [the Lord] keep him in perfect peace whose mind is stayed on you, because he trusts in you. Trust in the Lord forever, for the Lord God is an everlasting rock." The key is to keep our mind stayed on Him, not on shifting circumstances. You might have heard this adage: We may not know what the future holds, but we know Who holds the future.

Trust is the opposite of worry. We cannot trust and worry at the same time. We have to choose what we're going to keep our mind fixed upon. It's better to choose trust, because worry accomplishes nothing. Jesus posed this instructive question to His followers: "Can all your worries add a single moment to your life?" (Matthew 6:27, NLT).

During our son's slow recovery, I had abundant opportunities to choose between trust and worry. My husband and our son constantly faced those moment-by-moment choices too. It's easier to choose trust when we keep our eyes on Him.

One day, this verse came to our son three times while he lay confined in bed: "Be still, and know that I am God" (Psalm 46:10a). Physically, our son was already lying still. He recognized that God wanted him to be *spiritually* still and simply look up to Him. He later told me that he did a lot of thinking that day, pondering what God was doing in his life. When we are bedridden, we have a *lot* more time to think about God, and He has time to reveal Himself to us. I could see that God was connecting on a new level with our son.

Our son walked out of the hospital on the fortieth day. That number felt symbolic. I thought of Noah, who had to stay in the ark during forty continuous days of rain (Genesis 7:17). Jesus had emerged from the desert after forty days of temptation. They both endured forty-day trials with God's help.

After discharge from the hospital, it took weeks for our son to get off the high doses of narcotics he'd been prescribed to control his pain, which included fentanyl (up to fifty times stronger per gram than heroin, one hundred times stronger than morphine). He endured the rigors of narcotic withdrawal (not so different from what a heroin addict goes through if he doesn't get another fix). God brought him through all of that, too.

God *is* eminently trustworthy. Choose to place your full trust in Him every step of the way for the rest of your life's journey. God is with believers today, and He *will* be in all of our tomorrows, time without end.

13

___

Give Thanks

Ann Voskamp authored a best-selling memoir called *One Thousand Gifts*. When she was a young child, she encountered horrible loss. A sibling died in a tragic accident. Her toddler sister, while chasing a cat onto their family farm's driveway, was struck by a delivery truck. Ann later questioned whether there could be a God up in heaven and, *if* one existed, whether He could possibly be a good God, full of love and grace. Who can blame her?

Years later, after suffering anxiety, bitterness, fear, and fatigue, she began to wonder whether she could ever be joyful again. A friend challenged Ann to compile a list of one thousand things she could be thankful for. Ann began writing down everyday things she noticed and appreciated, like the jam on her toast, the scent of a florist's shop, or the cry of a blue jay in a spruce tree. She began to see that these were gifts from a loving, gracious God. On and on the list continued: warm cookies, crackling flames in the fireplace, moonlight shining down on pillows. Ann completed her goal of listing one thousand reasons to be thankful.

Ann continued to learn about gratitude, including this lesson: Being grateful for obviously good gifts was much easier than being grateful when tough things came her way. No matter how many reasons to be thankful we can name, loss still happens and pain still comes. Yet, *even then*, God wants us to have grateful hearts, *even when* sickness, injury, or suffering feel like a slap in the face from the Divine One.

Ann's seven-year-old son badly injured his hand when it got caught between whirring fan blades in the barn of their family farm. Each circulating blade measured two feet long and two pounds heavy. Ann drove him straight to the nearest emergency centre. Could she be grateful in that furnace of affliction? She thanked God for saving her son's hand. (Amazingly, he didn't even lose a single finger, although one broken, twisted finger required surgery.) She also expressed thanks for smaller matters, such as bandages and the availability of pain relief.

On the drive home, she heard on the news that another local farm boy, thirteen years old, had just died in an accident. She chose to be thankful that her family calamity, although serious, was not terminally serious.

Ann learned afresh through the fan-blade accident that God's grace could be found even in grief. God is so full of goodness, He can transfigure the ugliest of situations into something beautiful, just as He took the death of His Son Jesus on the cross and made that wretched suffering into the most achingly beautiful moment in all of history.

God wants us all to give thanks to Him—when the sun is shining and the sky is blue and all is well, but *also* when the fierce storms roll in. So many Bible verses command us to give thanks in *all* circumstances. Ephesians 5:20, for example, tells us to give thanks "always and for everything..." In 1 Thessalonians 5:16–18, we're instructed: "Rejoice always, pray without ceasing, give thanks in all circumstances; for this is the will of God in Christ Jesus for you." Psalm 136 repeats, over and over, that we should give thanks to the Lord.

Daniel understood the importance of being grateful to God. He prayed three times every day, always giving thanks to God no matter what (Daniel 6:10).

Jesus modelled an astounding ability to be grateful. He paused to thank God for the bread He was about to break at the Last Supper, knowing He would soon have to endure an agonizing death on the cross (1 Corinthians 11:23–24).

Not every biblical figure thanked God. Luke 17:11–18 tells the story of ten lepers coming to Jesus and asking Him for mercy. Jesus told them to present themselves to their priests. As they obediently went on their way, all of them were cleansed of leprosy. Only *one* of the ten returned to thank Jesus.

Let's choose to give thanks to our Healer. Even better, let's choose to thank God even before our full healing comes. While enduring sickness and suffering for a season, we can still thank God for life and breath and many other blessings.

The point of our thanksgiving is *not* to make God feel valued. God doesn't need our validation. God tells us to thank Him because He knows how much *we* will benefit from an attitude of gratitude.

You might recall one model of prayer structure we discussed, called ACTS. The "T" stands for thanksgiving. The positive nature of giving thanks during prayer offsets the negativity of confession and supplication (our lists of what's wrong with us and our circumstances). Thanksgiving allows us to focus on all the good things we can be grateful for. Offering specific thanks to God helps us to feel better.

Philippians 4:6–7 instructs us to not be anxious about anything, but to pray about everything, with *thanksgiving*. We must pray in a thankful spirit. If you often complain when you pray, make this the day that you resolve to break that habit. Begin punctuating your list of needs with frequent expressions of gratitude to God.

We can, for example, give thanks for what He has already done. The psalmist Asaph wrote: "I will remember the deeds of the Lord; yes, I will remember your wonders of old. I will ponder all your work, and meditate on your mighty deeds" (Psalm 77:11–12). Has God ever healed you (or a loved one) in the past? Pause right now to remember that and to thank Him.

One spring, my sister developed vision problems in her right eye. She lived in Afghanistan at the time. The first indication of something wrong was some obstruction of her vision. Then she observed an unusual halo surrounding her kitchen light. When she commented on these symptoms to her friend, an eye nurse, her friend insisted she go to the eye hospital in Kabul the next morning. After tests, the medical staff told my sister that the retina in her right eye was detaching. She needed an operation immediately or she could go blind within days. By God's grace, the optometrist had the telephone number of an ophthalmologist in Dubai that he had recently met. My sister flew out the next day. The ophthalmologist she consulted in Dubai arranged for a top eye surgeon to perform the operation the following day. Having surgery in a foreign country was scary, but my sister was amazed at how God had gone before her to order her steps. Although her vision was not completely restored in the affected eye, my sister is thankful for the measure of sight she retained. She was able to return to Afghanistan for many further years, overseeing her charitable organization.

I have decided to thank God after some of my own medical journeys.

In the late 1980s, whenever I styled my hair, a mole on my neck near my hairline would bleed a little. I ignored the issue at first, because the mole was small in diameter, the same brown colour throughout, and perfectly round, with no irregular edges. Except for the bleeding, it looked normal, even to my doctor husband. He suggested, however, that I see a doctor to have the mole removed and sent for analysis.

The lab results came back indicating the excised mole contained basal cell carcinoma. I was shocked and anxious when I learned that the innocent-looking mole had harboured skin cancer.

Even though the mole had been removed, I had to have some surrounding tissue removed in a second procedure performed by an oncologist who specialized in skin cancer. He made sure that an optimal surgical margin encircled the former mole site.

Both the dermatologist and the oncologist told me quite firmly that I would have to be careful about sun exposure for the rest of my life. Basal cell carcinoma quite commonly occurs in the elderly population.

I was still in my early thirties. Cancer cells showing up at that age did not bode well for the future of my skin.

The oncologist further told me there was no guarantee that he had removed every single cancer cell. He recommended that I have the site checked a few times that year and then annually thereafter (along with the rest of my skin).

After learning that the mole contained cancer cells, I looked for reasons to thank God. Why? Focusing on gratitude felt better than being overwhelmed with fear. Every time I thanked God for something, I felt less anxious. We can only feel one emotion in any particular moment. Every moment I spent thanking God was one less moment wasted on ruminating about further cancer in my future.

What did I thank God for back then? I was glad that I had the mole removed when I did. Had I waited longer, the carcinoma would have spread further and much more tissue would have had to be excised. I thanked God that I had been able to speedily see a dermatologist and then an oncologist who specialized in skin cancer. I thanked God that I live in a country that allows such great medical care at no personal cost. I was also very grateful that basal cell carcinoma is the least serious skin cancer.

As I continue to monitor my skin, I've found further reasons to be thankful. I've been careful about sun exposure in the decades following. My skin isn't as sun-damaged as it might otherwise have been. (I used to love tanning. I grew up in an era when a tan was considered a mark of healthy living. If that mole hadn't been cancerous, I would probably have kept on avidly tanning for years.) I'm thankful that I live in a country with four seasons, limiting days of heavy exposure to ultraviolet rays. When visiting tropical locations, I'm always grateful for shade.

I thank God that no further cancer has developed around the site of the removed mole, or anywhere else on my skin, over the decades. I've had other suspicious moles removed, but they turned out to be benign. I also thank God that various dermatologists over the years have been careful to treat any precancerous skin changes. When we go looking for reasons to be thankful, it's amazing how many we can find.

Lately, I've been thanking God, yet again, for healing me of the muscle disease that debilitated me more than half a century ago. I was just a child then, and I know I didn't thank Him very much at the time. In my adult years, I have, on occasion, poured out full-hearted thanksgiving—not just for the healing, but also for some related expressions of God's goodness.

In retrospect, I can see that many good things came out of the stretch of time I contended with illness as a child. I became a keen reader while in the hospital for several weeks. I hadn't been particularly interested in books before then. My sister went to our school library and signed out a book for me by British author Enid Blyton called *The Mountain of Adventure*. It was fantastic! I couldn't put it down. The book relieved my boredom and helped me forget my loneliness, immobility, and pain. I mentally travelled to a distant place, far away from my hospital bed, and lived a grand adventure alongside four daring British kids and their comical parrot, Kiki.

After I finished the book, my sister borrowed six more Blyton library books, all with the word "Adventure" in their titles. My parents then bought me *The River of Adventure*, which still sits on my bookshelf. I've given away many books over a lifetime, but *that* book will stay with me to my grave. Those delightful books cultivated in me an adventurous spirit. I developed a desire to travel out in the real world. I later did that extensively in my adult years. (I passed the one-hundred-country mark a while ago.)

After leaving the hospital, I remained weak and easily fatigued for months. Sad to still be physically limited, I compensated by signing out more books from the school library. Being transformed into an eager reader changed my life in a colossal way. Books educated me in a variety of subjects. I learned to read at a good clip. I developed the ability to absorb and remember what I was reading. This later made law school, which involved so much reading, easier for me than it was for many others. In my career, the large briefs I had to read before arguing cases in court didn't intimidate me. The senior lawyer I worked with assigned me most of his mega-files, some containing millions of documents. On days I didn't commute into the office, I made coffee, sat by the fireside on a comfy sofa, and read files for hours while the kids were at school—amazed that I was being paid to read.

Most importantly, it has never been a chore for me to read through the whole Bible, over and over again. As a result, I developed in-depth knowledge of many biblical subjects, including healing.

I've heard it said that one becomes a reader long before they become a writer. Reading nurtured in me a love of words, an appreciation of the beauty and utility of language. These days I write as passionately as I read.

I can now look back and thank God, *really thank Him*, for the many childhood weeks I spent in hospital, followed by further months of recovery. Without that stretch of sitting around so much, I might not have developed such a taste for reading. I might not have experienced the many roads that the enjoyment of reading later led me down. I can now see God's blessing shining brightly through my childhood season of sickness. He worked all things together for my good (Romans 8:28).

As you thank God for past healings, can you now see some good things that arose from any season of sickness, disability, or immobility? Thank God for whatever He accomplished in seasons of challenge.

What's happening in the present? Are you in need of healing now? Even if you haven't been healed yet, you can still find reasons to thank God. A friend named Jenny made a long list of reasons to be thankful while going through several weeks of radiation for breast cancer. She thanked God that the cancer was discovered early; it hadn't spread to the lymph nodes; the surgery to remove the breast lump wasn't extensive; she underwent treatment fairly quickly after diagnosis; her circumstances did not require chemotherapy; she had excellent oncologists; she could afford to take time off work; she had a support network of family members and friends; and she had many people praying for her. It's one thing to be thankful after treatment achieves remission, but it's quite another to be thankful while still in the midst of testing and treatment, pain and fatigue, facing an uncertain future.

We can give thanks on behalf of sick loved ones, noticing what God is doing for them, even while they're still suffering. Offering gratitude to God can strengthen us and cheer us up. It can help to sustain faith, trust, and hope.

I encourage you to thank God for His healing work in the past and for all good things that flowed out of any season of illness, injury, or disability. Also thank Him in the present, *whatever* you are going through. Then thank Him for promising to be with you in the future, every step of the way, from this life right through to the next. Ann Voskamp's memoir demonstrates that gratitude *can* become a daily habit. Let's challenge ourselves to be grateful in the best of days *and* the worst of days.

14

PRAISE HIM

I confess I'm not always spiritually positive. During the long hospitalizations of loved ones, I've sometimes left bedsides feeling depleted and discouraged. I have trudged outside, hoping that some fresh air would revive both body and soul. Alone with God, my first instinct has often been to cry out to Him in pain and petition. I've wanted relief. I've wanted circumstances to change. Above all, I've wanted a loved one to be healed.

As I've pounded the pavement in prayerful lament, I've sometimes sensed God telling me to *praise* Him, not just petition Him. I used to wonder how I could praise God while a loved one languished in the hospital. How could I worship while they suffered and struggled (and I struggled too)? Yet on many such occasions, I couldn't mistake God's nudge, deep within, to offer up to Him my praise. During my husband's hospitalization for a brain bleed, I wrote in my journal on day five: "God has been telling me to praise Him."

God has helped me with the process of praising Him in the midst of pain. One day, I left my husband's hospital room, feeling spent. Sam hadn't been very communicative that day. I'd sat by his bedside for hours, lonely and sad. I walked downstairs with a heavy heart. As I crossed the hospital lobby, I encountered a small choir of men singing the chorus of a favourite Christmas carol, "Gloria in Excelsis Deo." I felt like a warm, comforting cloak had encircled my weary shoulders as I listened to the familiar chorus. Praise welled up in my heart. Isaiah 61:3 foretold that Jesus would give us many things, including a "garment of praise instead of a faint spirit…"

Paul wrote: "… let us continually offer up a sacrifice of praise to God…" (Hebrews 13:15). The word "continually" suggests we should praise God in every circumstance, good or bad. The word "sacrifice" indicates that the praise will cost us something. At times, praise comes naturally to us. Other times, it seems counterintuitive, and it requires great effort. The sacrifice of praise, offered up in tough times, differs from the kind of exuberant praise that spontaneously spills out of our spirit when all is wonderfully right with our world. Psalm 34:1 affirms that we are to praise God in the sunshine *and* in the storm: "I will praise the Lord at all times…" Thanksgiving primarily focuses on *what* God has done for us. Praise focuses more on *who* God is.

I have inwardly praised Him during some very dark hours. I have forced myself to praise Him even when, on various occasions, loved ones were sick almost to the point of death, when praise was the *last* thing I felt like doing. I have praised Him silently while watching them weep in despair, when pain sabotaged their bodies, when the relief of morphine ended after measured infusions ran dry, when overwhelming pain then seized them again, and at points when everything seemed to be going wrong.

I learned that praise made a difference. After moments of quiet praise, a loved one would fall peacefully asleep or sit up to eat the lunch they had earlier pushed away. God loves praise and responds to it. God is always worthy of praise.

We can praise Him directly, but we can also express praise in the way we talk *about* Him with others. Most of us have no trouble praising a favourite author, actor, artist, chef, athlete, or musician. We are so quick to speak words of praise to (or about) the humans we admire. How much quicker we should be to praise Almighty God!

Praise releases God's power. Jehoshaphat, King of Judah, understood the power of praise. In 2 Chronicles 20, we read about a massive foreign army coming against Jehoshaphat. The marauding army outnumbered Judah's army. God told Jehoshaphat that He would win the battle for him. Instead of sending experienced soldiers to the battlefront, Jehoshaphat sent singers to the front of the line (v. 21). Can you imagine that extraordinary scene? The singers praised God in advance of victory. They sang about God's enduring love, confusing the enemy soldiers, who began to fight one another (vv. 22–23). By simply praising God, Jehoshaphat's army defeated their stronger opponents without lifting a sword. Let's never underestimate the power of praise. Instead, let's praise God on the battlefront.

The prophet Jeremiah recognized the connection between praise and healing. He wrote: "Heal me, Lord, and I will be healed; save me and I will be saved, for you are the one I praise" (Jeremiah 17:14, NIV). Jeremiah's praise preceded his healing.

Like thanksgiving, praise is for *our* benefit. When I praise Him for His steadfast love, I create the opportunity to focus on that incomparable love. Fresh awareness of His love can then warm every cell in my body. When I praise Him for His goodness, I then notice His goodness all around me. During a hospital visit, His goodness might show up in an elevator quick to arrive (a miracle in a busy hospital), or a doctor willing to take time to answer questions. If I don't praise Him, I might be oblivious to such blessings. When I praise His unrivalled power, He might demonstrate it by a fever resolved, or perhaps a loved one getting out of bed to walk for the first time in weeks. When I praise Him for His mercy, a winter day might go by without ice or wind or snow, and my walk through the visitors' parking lot might surprisingly refresh me.

Praise shifts our focus onto Him. The world can seem lighter and brighter with each good thought we have about Him. Praise can elevate our mood, reminding us of all that is right about God, taking our attention away from all that seems wrong about our situation. Praise can take our minds off sickness, symptoms, suffering, pending surgery, potential complications, actual complications, and all the what-ifs. It can drive fear and anxiety out of our minds. Praise can catalyze hope, comfort, peace, and even joy, at times when such states hardly seem possible. It can renew our energy, helping us to keep on keeping on, perhaps with clearer vision of a better future.

Earlier, we discussed a prayer model known by the acronym ACTS. The "A" stands for adoration, one facet of praise.

The Lord's Prayer, which Jesus taught His disciples, fittingly begins: "… Our Father in heaven, hallowed be your name" (Matthew 6:9, NIV). Synonyms of the word "hallowed" include "praised" and "revered." Before we pray about needs, we can meditate on His greatness. Praise and adoration can flow from the love, respect, and awe we feel for Him. Reviewing some chapters in this book (about God's power, character, glory, giving nature, and willingness to heal) can remind you of many reasons to praise Him.

We can prayerfully recite psalms of praise in moments when we cannot come up with our own free-form expression of adoration. One psalmist exclaimed: "Praise is due to you, O God…" (Psalm 65:1). Other psalmists wrote: "Praise the Lord, for the Lord is good…" (Psalm 135:3) and "Let everything that has breath praise the Lord!" (Psalm 150:6a). Are you still breathing? Then praise Him.

Praise comes (relatively) easily when we offer it up to God for others. After all, *we* are still (hopefully) able to sleep, eat, exercise, take breaks, and carry on with some normal routines. Praise is toughest when *we* are sick, in pain, exhausted, or despairing.

I remember all too well my confrontation with the nasty bacteria *C. difficile*, which attacked my gut like terrorists bent on destruction. I eventually stopped eating and quickly lost several pounds. I struggled to keep hydrated, one tiny sip at a time, but even a few swallows of weak tea, or a spoonful or two of clear soup, made me rush to the bathroom. Although the bacterial assault had weakened me, the urgency of reaching the bathroom propelled my feeble legs into action. I sat in the bathroom for long stretches of time, day and night, passing mostly water while I shivered and shook. The vicious bacteria kept multiplying. I didn't have the strength to phone, text, or email to rally prayer warriors. My husband, still recovering from his brain bleed, didn't have much strength either, but I finally let him take me to the hospital. I had to overcome my fear of being nowhere near a toilet for that fifteen-minute drive. I received an immediate sigmoidoscopy and the diagnosis of *C. difficile*. Several weeks of treatment began. I later learned that, had I not received timely treatment, the severe level of illness I'd been fighting could have become fatal.

Even during the bleakest days, I sensed God asking me, deep within my soul, to praise Him. I summoned up the last fragments of inner strength to do so, even though His request seemed ridiculous. At times, my praise felt empty. It took herculean effort, but it was worth it. Prayerful praise somehow sustained me when I couldn't eat, or sleep, or read, or when I threw up my medication. Praise poured surprising comfort into me when I chose to enter into it. It multiplied the particles of faith I had left faster than the bacteria could multiply. Very few people knew I was sick, so cards and flowers were not arriving, but He was there with me. He dwells in the midst of praise. His presence was enough. His healing power came down.

After years of learning such lessons, it's more natural to me now to praise God whenever my world is falling apart. Once we've experienced the power of praise, it becomes a more normal response.

Most often I praise God in prayer, but we can also *sing* praise. Psalm 135:3 suggests: "Praise the Lord, for the Lord is good; sing to his name..." Similarly, Psalm 150 encourages us to praise God with song. I sometimes sing praise music to myself when I'm feeling weak or weary.

Let's remember to keep on praising God *after* His healing power has come down, as these people did:

> *Jesus left there and went along the Sea of Galilee. Then he went up on a mountainside and sat down. Great crowds came to him, bringing the lame, the blind, the crippled, the mute and many others, and laid them at his feet; and he healed them. The people*

were amazed when they saw the mute speaking, the crippled made
well, the lame walking and the blind seeing. And they praised the
God of Israel.

Matthew 15:29–31, NIV

God spared David's life and healed him. Afterward, David wrote: "Sing praises to the Lord, O you his saints, and give thanks to his holy name" (Psalm 30:4).

Let's praise God, in sickness and in health, while waiting for healing, and then again after it has come. Joel 2:26 states: "…praise the name of the Lord your God, who has dealt wondrously with you." God, and God alone, is worthy of our worship.

A few months after Sam's brain bleed hospitalization, and after medication helped vanquish the *C. difficile* in my body, I often sang to myself songs of praise. God had been so good. He had helped us both on our roads to recovery. Around that time, I began writing this book as one further way to praise God.

15

OBEY HIM

If you've been taking care of your body, spending time in His Word, choosing faith, trusting Him, praying, and offering Him gratitude and praise, then you've already taken many steps of obedience.

Moses wrote:

> *… If you will diligently listen to the voice of the Lord your God, and do that which is right in his eyes, and give ear to his commandments and keep all his statutes, I [the Lord] will put none of the diseases on you that I put on the Egyptians, for I am the Lord, your healer.*
>
> Exodus 15:26

Moses later told the Israelites:

> *You shall serve the Lord your God, and he will bless your bread and your water, and I [the Lord] will take sickness away from among you. None shall miscarry or be barren in your land; I [the Lord] will fulfill the number of your days.*
>
> Exodus 23:25–26

On yet another occasion, Moses stated:

... because you listen to these rules and keep and do them, the Lord
your God will keep with you the covenant and the steadfast love
that he swore to your fathers... And the Lord will take away from
you all sickness, and none of the evil diseases of Egypt, which you
knew, will he inflict on you...

Deuteronomy 7:12, 15

In Deuteronomy 28, Moses further expounded on the positive connection between obedience and blessings (which include good health).

In a later era, Solomon advised: "... fear the Lord and shun evil.
This will bring health to your body and nourishment to your bones"
(Proverbs 3:7–8, NIV).

In the New Testament era, Jesus linked obedience with healing.
For example, He told a parable about a sower who sowed the Word of
God into various lives. Some received it, took it to heart, and lived by
it; others did not. Jesus declared that *if* a person would see, hear, and
understand the Word of God, and "turn" (from sin to repentance and
obedience), *then* God "would heal them" (Matthew 13:15).

Obedience isn't always easy. At times, we will struggle to obey
Him. At times, we will fail. God wants to help us. The apostle Paul
told the Christians at Philippi: "Work hard to show the results of
your salvation, obeying God with deep reverence and fear. For God
is working in you, giving you the desire and the power to do what
pleases him" (Philippians 2:12c–13, NLT).

Sometimes the obedience required of us is directly linked to our
quest for healing. In the Old Testament, we read about Naaman, an Ar-
amean military commander, who had leprosy (2 Kings 5:1–14). Elisha, a
Jewish prophet, told Naaman to wash himself in the Jordan River seven
times. At first, Naaman resisted Elisha's directive, probably wondering
what good it would do, but later he decided to follow it. Afterward, his
skin became as smooth as the skin of a young boy.

In Mark 3:1–6, we learn about a man with a deformed hand who
met Jesus in a synagogue on the Sabbath. Jesus told the man to stretch
out his withered hand. *After* the man obediently extended his hand, it

was restored, becoming as normal as the other hand. You might be thinking that this stretching forth was an easy act of obedience. Not so. The
disabled man had to obey Jesus in the presence of some Pharisees, who
belonged to a Jewish sect known for strictly upholding religious laws.
Jesus was aware of the "hardness of heart" of those religious leaders
(Mark 3:5). By complying with what Jesus asked him to do, the man aid-
ed and abetted Jesus in flouting the Sabbath law, upsetting the religious
leaders who thereafter plotted to destroy Jesus. The healed man risked
being ostracized, or even persecuted, in his synagogue community.

John 9:1–7 provides another example of healing following active
obedience. Jesus mixed saliva with mud and placed it on the eyes of
a blind man. Jesus then told the man to go and wash in the pool of
Siloam. Jesus could have fully healed that blind man right on the spot,
but He made the man take a step of obedience. The man couldn't see
until he obediently washed the mud off his eyes in the designated
pool. (You can visit that pool today, in Jerusalem, in the City of David
archaeological site.)

Jesus told many ailing people to rise up and walk. They were
healed in the process of doing what He told them to do.

Sometimes healing occurs after obedience to a general biblical
command. Did you know, for example, that God connects helping the
poor with the blessing of being healed? Psalm 41 states: "Blessed is the
one who considers the poor!... The Lord sustains him on his sickbed;
in his illness you [the Lord] restore him to full health" (vv. 1, 3).

Isaiah 58 links healing with obedient willingness to go beyond
mere religious ritual, into the higher realm of showing caring concern
for others. In that chapter, we learn that God wasn't impressed with
the fasting that the people of Israel engaged in. The people sought to
appear righteous while they kept on living in wrong relationship with
both God and man. God spoke, in response to that behaviour, through
the prophet Isaiah:

> *Is this not the kind of fasting I have chosen: to loose the chains of
> injustice and untie the cords of the yoke, to set the oppressed free*

*and break every yoke? Is it not to share your food with the hungry
and to provide the poor wanderer with shelter—when you see the
naked, to clothe them, and not to turn away from your own flesh
and blood? Then your light will break forth like the dawn, and
your healing will quickly appear; then your righteousness will go
before you, and the glory of the Lord will be your rear guard. Then
you will call, and the Lord will answer; you will cry for help, and
He will say "Here am I."*

Isaiah 58:6–9a, NIV

In contrast to the healing power that obedience releases, disobedience to God's commands can have a destructive impact on our health. Deuteronomy 28 warns about the negative connection between disobedience and disease.

Similarly, Leviticus 26:14–16b cautions:

… if you do not listen to me [the Lord] or obey all these commands, and if you break my covenant by rejecting my decrees, treating my regulations with contempt, and refusing to obey my commands, I will punish you. I will bring sudden terrors upon you—wasting diseases and burning fevers that will cause your eyes to fail and your life to ebb away. (NLT)

Not all illness arises from disobeying God's precepts. That point must be made loud and clear. We might get sick because of other reasons: dysfunctional genes we inherited (through no fault of our own), or because of some virus we catch (through no fault of our own), or because the world we live in has become polluted and contaminated (by humanity through the ages). If someone we know gets sick, we must *never* assume God has inflicted that sickness, or that the person has been disobedient. But *sometimes* sickness *is* the result of disobedience. We must judge ourselves in that regard if we become sick. (I repeat: It is not our job to judge others.)

David understood that sometimes sin and sickness are connected: "When I refused to confess my sin, my body wasted away, and I groaned all day long. Day and night your [the Lord's] hand of discipline was heavy on me. My strength evaporated like water in the summer heat" (Psalm 32:3–4, NLT). Later in that same psalm, David talked about how he finally confessed all his sins to God.

In another psalm, David wrote:

> *O Lord, don't rebuke me in your anger or discipline me in your*
> *rage!… Because of your anger, my whole body is sick; my health*
> *is broken because of my sins. My guilt overwhelms me—it is a*
> *burden too heavy to bear. My wounds fester and stink because of*
> *my foolish sins [including adultery and murder]. I am bent over*
> *and racked with pain. All day long I walk around filled with grief.*
> *A raging fever burns within me, and my health is broken. I am*
> *exhausted and completely crushed… My heart beats wildly, my*
> *strength fails, and I am going blind. My loved ones and friends*
> *stay away, fearing my disease… I am on the verge of collapse,*
> *facing constant pain. But I confess my sins; I am deeply sorry for*
> *what I have done… Do not abandon me, O Lord. Do not stand at*
> *a distance, my God. Come quickly to help me, O Lord my savior.*
>
> Psalm 38:1, 3–8, 10-11, 17–18, 21–22, NLT

The prophet Jeremiah connected sickness to sin (particularly rebellion against God). In Jeremiah 8:22, Jeremiah asked: "Is there no balm in Gilead? Is there no physician there? Why then has the health of the daughter of my people not been restored?" The answer can be found in the surrounding verses, in which Jeremiah discusses the disobedience of God's people.

Although the death of Jesus on the cross has removed from us the curse of the Old Testament law, disobedience can still separate us from the blessings God wants to bestow.

Jesus *sometimes* made a connection between sin and sickness (but not always). On some occasions, after He had healed people, Jesus instructed them to go and sin no more, implying that their physical ailment had been related to their sin. For example, after Jesus healed the lame man at the Pool of Bethesda, He told him to stop sinning, or something worse might happen to him (John 5:14). In both Matthew 9:1–7 and Mark 2:1–11, we learn that Jesus forgave the sins of a paralytic before He healed him.

If we dare to reject God, or to treat His ways with contempt, we cannot expect to receive His love, mercy, and grace. If we don't readily confess any disobedience, we cannot expect Him to hear our petitions for healing. Ignoring known sin creates a barrier between God and us. We are one simple confession away from God's gracious forgiveness, if we genuinely want His help in turning from our sinful behaviour.

I've had to humble myself and confess my sins to God, in certain times of sickness, when I sensed the Spirit nudging my conscience over a particular matter. When my health quickly and seriously deteriorated due to *C. difficile* in my bowel, God spoke to me about a particular attitude of my heart. God pressed that issue while the painful *C. difficile* bacteria wreaked havoc with my digestive system. That wrong attitude didn't cause my sickness, but God used my season of sickness to correct it.

I encourage you to seek the Lord today and deal with any sin that separates you from His holy presence. Resolve to be more obedient to His commands.

The prophet Amos 5:6 declared: "Seek the Lord and live…"

16

Choose Hope

On a few occasions, my family spent time on a friend's yacht in the idyllic British Virgin Islands. During the day, we island-hopped, swam, and snorkelled. At night, the captain fastened the boat to a mooring ball. One night, all of the mooring balls in the bay were taken, so our captain had to use the yacht's anchor. Of course, *that* was the night that a tropical storm blew in.

After midnight, I lay awake, listening to the hostile wind, feeling the yacht bobbing wildly. I wondered if the anchor, hooked into the sandy seabed, would remain secure, able to stop the boat from breaking loose and drifting out to sea. The wind and waves were likely much more tumultuous beyond our sheltered bay. I finally fell asleep, *hoping* that the anchor would hold us. I woke up after the storm, relieved to discover that the anchor had kept us tethered to the seabed. All was well.

In the tempests of life, we need a strong and steady anchor. In Hebrew 6:18–19, Paul instructed us to "hold fast to the hope set before us," because hope is "a sure and steadfast anchor of the soul…" Hope anchors us to the presence, power, and promises of Almighty God. I'm glad that I can anchor my hope in my steadfast God, not in my shifting, sometimes stormy circumstances.

The Old Testament figure Job endured many severe trials, including health issues. Yet Job could say: "Though he [God] slay me, I will hope in him" (Job 13:15a). I've personalized that verse and have often spoken it to God in my prayers: Though You seem to be slaying me, yet will I hope in You.

In Psalm 43:5, we see that David sometimes felt very discouraged, "cast down," and in "turmoil." Instead of staying in that state, David chose to hope in God. David believed he would again have reason to praise Him.

Hope and faith become intertwined, like the chain links attaching an anchor to a vessel. They support each other. If we choose to have faith, then it's much easier to also have hope, and vice versa. Faith and hope are two of the three things that can remain strong and secure even when everything else seems to be failing (1 Corinthians 13:13).

Abraham modelled both faith and hope. God told Abraham and Sarah that they would become parents, despite their advanced age. Their descendants would be as numerous as the grains of sand on the seashore and the stars in the sky:

> *Against all hope, Abraham in hope believed and so became the*
> *father of many nations, just as it had been said to him …Without*
> *weakening in his faith, he faced the fact that his body was as*
> *good as dead—since he was about a hundred years old—and*
> *that Sarah's womb was also dead. Yet he did not waver through*
> *unbelief regarding the promise of God, but was strengthened in his*
> *faith and gave glory to God, being fully persuaded that God had*
> *power to do what he had promised.*
>
> Romans 4:18–21, NIV

Choosing hope matters.

Years ago, our young teenage son was hospitalized for a few weeks because of abdominal inflammation. Not allowed to eat for eleven days, he received a liquid nutritional supplement intravenously. He lost weight and grew weak. The doctors prescribed six medications, then bluntly recommended immediate surgery.

Our son swallowed barium for a necessary radiological test. The doctors couldn't order a pre-surgery CT scan or perform surgery until all of that barium fully flushed out of his bowel. The doctors kept commenting that the barium was taking an unusually long time to clear our son's system. Perhaps God was up to something.

Around that time, a teacher visited our son in the hospital and told him that his eighth-grade graduating class had elected him to be their valedictorian. My husband and I told the teacher that our son, still ill, was slated to undergo surgery around the same date as the graduation ceremony. Then, although it seemed ridiculous, we asked the teacher to give our son a few days to consider the invitation to speak. The honour of being selected valedictorian gave our son something positive to focus on.

I didn't think that our son had the strength to write a speech, but he was surprisingly enthusiastic, even though he knew he might not be able to attend his graduation. He dared to hope he'd be well enough to give the speech, even though the medical team continued to advise us that surgery was imminent.

Our son asked us to bring a laptop to the hospital. He began working on his talk while the barium stubbornly lingered in his body. When he discussed different ideas for his speech with me, he almost seemed like his usual self. I valued such upbeat moments, because he'd gone through low moods in previous days.

Our son even wanted us to rent him a tuxedo for his grad night. I brought a tape measure into the hospital to determine his tuxedo size. This drew ire from one of the senior doctors, who thought my behaviour was irresponsible. That doctor was certain our son would develop disappointment and depression when he couldn't attend his graduation ceremony to deliver his speech. The same doctor told me to stop discussing the speech and to instead emotionally prepare my son for the surgery and its aftermath.

I carefully considered the doctor's advice, which I had to admit was reasonable. Yet I continued to strongly sense God prompting me to help our son prepare his speech. Many times, my son and I prayed together that he would somehow be able to give the valedictory address. I kept asking him if he wanted to do it. He said that he did. (As a fallback scenario, I knew that another student could read our son's speech on grad night. I never told our son that, because I didn't want to dilute his hope.)

In the days that it took our son's body to flush out the barium, his condition improved, surprising all the doctors. Our son received the go-ahead to eat again. His digestive system began normalizing. The medical team began questioning the urgency of the surgery they'd been advocating.

Our son received a few-hours pass, allowing him to leave the hospital to attend his graduation. A kind nurse capped the intravenous line that fed into one of his central arteries, cautioning him not to disturb the capped line. Our son then dressed up in his debonair tuxedo. As I later watched our son walk into the school gymnasium with the procession of his fellow graduates, I could barely believe we were there.

Near the end of the evening, our son walked up on stage and stood up in front of hundreds of people (his fellow students, their families, his teachers, and his principal). He was still quite weak and wobbly on his feet. He'd only been eating for a few days and was much under his normal weight. But he looked great in his black tuxedo. He spoke clearly, with a strength and vigour that belied the rough hospitalization he'd endured for almost three weeks. Most teachers and classmates hadn't seen him in all that time. Many cried unabashedly, their tears mixing with their cheers. The speech was a great success. Our son even cracked some jokes that generated much laughter. Can you believe that our son even had the energy to spend time at the grad dance, celebrating with his friends? That was far beyond what we had imagined and prayed for. God's palpable presence that night helped the three of us to sustain our faith and hope in God's ability to restore health. Our son was under doctor's orders to return to the hospital before midnight. After he was settled in his bed, the nursing team gathered around to hear about his evening.

Having witnessed our son's dramatic recovery in the days just before grad night, and after hearing that he did deliver his speech, the medical team decided the next day not to proceed with surgery at that time. Instead, our son was soon discharged from hospital.

(Our son didn't have surgery for another nine years. In the meantime, God gave him victory over occasional periods of internal inflammation, one flare-up at a time. Our son eventually chose to have surgery, in a preferable period of peak health, at the stage of young adult life that he thought was most opportune.)

Some say they don't want to get their hopes up in case they get disappointed. They question: What if they hope and pray for healing and it doesn't happen? What if it doesn't happen in the timing, manner, and degree they've hoped for?

I look at hope differently. What happens if I *do* receive the restoration I'm praying for? What if my health at least improves? What if I'm *not* disappointed? Romans 5:5 assures me that those who hope in the Lord will never be disappointed. Someday I will arrive in heaven. My hope that I will spend eternity with Him, in a resurrected body immortal and indestructible, far outweighs my hope for healing in this temporal world. It's not a lesser hope. Hope for healing in this lifetime and hope for our ultimate destiny in heaven can run *together*, simultaneously, on parallel tracks. Both hopes can peacefully co-exist. A drawing done with proper perspective will show parallel tracks, such as train tracks or car tracks, meeting together at the distant horizon. Our side-by-side tracks, of two distinct hopes, will also meet at our last earthly horizon when this life passes into the next.

I have therefore firmly settled in my mind that I will never be disappointed after praying for healing. I may encounter days of struggle and sorrow, but I need not abandon hope. *Wherever* and *whenever*, a good outcome awaits me, here *or* there.

If we're praying for others, we need not worry about whether they will be healed. We can pray for them. We can also encourage them to keep on praying for themselves. We can challenge them to stir up their own hope. The outcome of it all is not our responsibility. Being a positive part of the process *is* our responsibility, especially if someone asks for our prayers. If we remain hopeful, we might succeed in fostering hope in them, for both healing here and heaven later.

When our son was still recovering in the hospital, one of my brothers visited. He told our son that God had great things in store for him. He believed that our son would get up out of the hospital bed and run again (a meaningful thing to say, because my son excelled at track and had won many races over the years). My brother's words generated hope in our son, who did get out of that hospital bed. He did run again. He kept on running. In football tryouts back in high school, he clocked in as the fastest runner out of the seventy-three guys hoping to make the team. He still runs sometimes, for exercise and for pleasure. I think of my brother's words when I see on social media that our son has been on a run. I also think of these words, penned by the prophet Isaiah: "… those who hope in the Lord will renew their strength. They will soar on wings like eagles. They will run and not grow weary, they will walk and not be faint" (Isaiah 40:31, NIV). These words have special meaning to those of us who have spent long days unable to get out of a sickbed.

Medical science has verified the power of hope as it pertains to healing outcomes. Studies have shown that patients who expect a positive outcome do better than those who don't. Optimism (similar to hope) benefits their mental health, coping skills, health-related quality of life, health-related behaviours, physical health outcomes, and longevity.[32]

The placebo effect also proves the power of hope. In clinical trials, some patients take the real medicine that's being studied, and others take sugar pills called placebos. Neither the patients nor the doctors know which patients are taking the actual medicine and which are receiving the placebo. Most clinical studies find that there is significant health improvement in as many as 35–45 percent of the patients who take the placebo pills. This shows that the hope of getting better has a positive impact on health.[33] If such hope in medication has power, imagine how much more powerful our hope in God must be.

Yet some have lost all hope that they can be physically healed. In 2016, with public support, the government of Canada passed a law permitting medically assisted death. (Those who opposed it called it medically assisted suicide.) Adults who chronically suffer with a medical condition leading to death can, within certain guidelines, ask a doctor to assist in ending their lives. Our lawmakers are now considering broader inclusion for doctor-assisted death for patients who: have chronic medical conditions that are not terminal; suffer mental health issues; are not yet adults; or do not have the capacity to seek assisted death for themselves (if a caregiver initiates the process). Other countries have extended the die-on-demand right to such patients.

God has set both life and death before us. God counsels us to choose life:

> *I [the Lord] call heaven and earth to witness against you today,*
> *that I have set before you life and death… Therefore choose life,*
> *that you and your offspring may live, loving the Lord your God,*
> *obeying his voice and holding fast to him, for he is your life and*
> *length of days …*
> Deuteronomy 30:19–20

If we have hope, we can choose life, no matter how greatly we suffer. We can do this if the source *and* the object of our hope is our mighty God. Paul encouraged us: "Let us hold unswervingly to the hope we profess, for he [the Lord] who promised is faithful" (Hebrews 10:23, NIV). Psalm 71:14 talks about hoping "continually."

The very first book of the Bible queries: "Is anything too hard for the Lord?" (Genesis 18:14a, NIV). Earlier in Genesis, we're told that God created the entire universe and everything in it, including humankind. Pause to reflect on that afresh and then reconsider the question: Is anything too hard for the Lord? I don't think so. We can safely anchor our hope in our all-powerful God, and in His love, mercy, and grace. Hope in God is much more potent than mere optimism or wishful thinking.

God never changes. What He has done before, He can do again. Malachi 3:6 records: "For I the Lord do not change..." Hebrews 13:8 advises: "Jesus Christ is the same yesterday and today and forever." Everything else in our lives is subject to change. Our health is subject to change. Sometimes it changes for the worse, but it can change again for the better.

We don't need to lose hope as we age. While our bodies will eventually decline to some degree, we might be surprised that aspects of our health might improve as we get older. On a recent visit to my optometrist, I was told my distance vision has improved. After my father's back-to-back heart attacks in his late sixties, he stopped smoking, began to walk more, and ate a better diet. He became healthier in his seventies than he had been in his fifties and sixties.

Hope in God must be active, not passive. Hope can *move* us to pray, praise, meditate on God's words, seek help, and do whatever else we can do to create positive change in our health. Hope creates energy so that we can do *something* rather than *nothing*. In response to our hope, and the positive activities that hope motivates, God Himself also moves. When He moves on our behalf, great things happen.

There's no such thing as "too much" hope in God. The apostle Paul declared that God is able to do exceedingly and abundantly more than we can ever dare to ask or think, dream, or desire (Ephesians 3:20). Paul stated that God will meet every one of our needs through His riches in Christ Jesus (Philippians 4:19). He further stated that we Christians should, by the power of the Holy Spirit, "abound in hope" (Romans 15:13).

Let us not be overwhelmed by the severity of our health problem(s). When God is for us, it doesn't matter what has come against us (Romans 8:31). The force who is on our side is greater than any forces assailing us. All things are possible with God (Mark 10:27). God can heal us in this life and He can raise us up to be with Him after we die.

God loves us and has good plans for us. Jeremiah 29:11 records: "For I know the plans I have for you, declares the Lord, plans for welfare and not for evil, to give you a future and a hope." God wants to bless those who hope in Him, not harm them.

Choose to hope in God! Like David, let Him know: "My hope is in you" (Psalm 39:7b). Hope with purpose and purpose to hope. Surround yourself with others who will encourage your hope. Fill your mind with God's hope-inspiring words. Let hope firmly anchor your soul, no matter how fiercely the tempest rages.

17

CALL ON HIS NAME

I have told you about the small plane that wrote two white-smoke words across a Florida sky: Trust Jesus. We have already considered the first word. Now let's focus on the second word, the exquisite name of Jesus.

As I stood in a hospital corridor and prayed while our son underwent emergency surgery, I kept inwardly repeating both words. When fatigue set in, I shortened my refrain to one word: Jesus. "Jesus, Jesus" my heart called out in those hours of uncertainty. God mercifully spared our son's life that terrible night. I kept calling on the name of Jesus for the duration of the long hospitalization that ensued.

Jesus: Name above all names. The name at which every knee will bow. The name that can vanquish any foe, including disease and even death. That name is not just a personal identifier. The name of Jesus contains great power.

In Hebrew, Jesus is translated as Yeshua, which means "God saves." It also means "God heals." When Jesus lived here on earth, the Jews believed that saving and healing were inseparable concepts.[34] They had no trouble believing that a God who was powerful enough to save could also heal. The name Yeshua evoked that dual power.

Jesus was well aware of the power contained in His name. He told His followers:

> *Again I say to you, if two of you agree on earth about anything they*
> *ask, it will be done for them by my Father in heaven. For where two*
> *or three are gathered in my name, there am I among them.*
>
> Matthew 18:19–20

Just before His death, Jesus told His followers: "Whatever you ask *in my name*, this will I do, that the Father may be glorified in the Son. If you ask me anything *in my name*, I will do it" (John 14:13–14).

Jesus further advised: "… I chose you and appointed you so that you might go and bear fruit—fruit that will last—and so that whatever you ask *in my name* the Father will give you" (John 15:16, NIV).

Yet again, Jesus stated:

> *Truly, truly, I say to you, whatever you ask the Father in my*
> *name, he will give it to you. Until now you have asked nothing in*
> *my name. Ask, and you will receive, that your joy may be full.*
>
> John 16:23b–24

Jesus repeated the instruction to pray in His name four times in one of His last conversations with His disciples. Why? When we pray in the name of Jesus, we come before the Father on the merit of what Jesus has done, *not* on the basis of our own merit. We don't approach Father God on the footing that we've been a believer for decades. Serving as a pastor, missionary, or Sunday School teacher doesn't earn us special standing with Him. No, we approach Almighty God purely on the basis of what His Son did for us on the cross. You and I kneel at the foot of the cross as equals, sinners saved by grace.

The followers of Jesus learned a lesson about the power of His name not long after He ascended. A man, crippled from birth, approached two of Jesus' disciples, Peter and John, and asked them for money. Peter responded: "… I have no silver and gold, but what I do have I give to you. *In the name* of Jesus Christ of Nazareth, rise up and walk!" (Acts 3:6). Peter then took the man's hand and raised him up. The man's feet and ankles became immediately strong. "And leaping up, he stood and began to walk, and entered the temple with them, walking and leaping and praising God" (Acts 3:8).

Soon after, Peter explained the miracle to the crowd:

> *By faith in the name of Jesus, this man whom you see and know was made strong. It is Jesus' name and the faith that comes through him that has given this complete healing to him, as you can all see.*
>
> Acts 3:16, NIV

John also referred to the potent name of Jesus:

> *Dear friends, if our hearts do not condemn us, we have confidence before God and receive from him anything we ask, because we obey his commands and do what pleases him. And this is his command: to believe in the name of his Son, Jesus Christ, and to love one another as he commanded us.*
>
> 1 John 3:21–23, NIV

Christians down through the ages have continued to value the name of Jesus. A majestic old hymn was titled "All Hail the Power of Jesus' Name." We, too, can believe in and revere the wonder-working name of Jesus.

Author Andrew Murray made an arresting point in his book on prayer. He posited that the extent of the dominion that Jesus has over our whole lives would affect the measure of the power that His name releases when we use it in our prayers. Murray further asserted that we must be willing to bear the name of Jesus in the company of others before we can use its full power in our prayers.[35] If we try to use the name of Jesus in our prayers the way a magician would use the word "abracadabra," we will likely be disappointed.

Healing stories often involve people calling out on the name of Jesus. Stormie Omartian, for example, called out on the name of Jesus when her appendix ruptured, spreading infection through her abdomen. In times of pain, the two syllables in His name are sometimes all we can utter. Yet those two syllables can grant access to the mighty healing power of God.

Even many non-Christians have come to see the power in the name of Jesus. Muslims believe that Jesus, called Isa in the Quran, was a great prophet. On that basis, Muslims might be interested in talking about Jesus. Some will allow themselves to be prayed for in the name of Jesus.

My sister worked in Afghanistan for more than two decades. She prayed in person for many Muslim women and their family members to be healed in the name of Jesus (Isa). God healed some of them. While visiting my sister in Afghanistan, a few young girls approached us near their village, told us about their health needs, and allowed us to pray for them in the name of Jesus. I will never forget that experience.

Brother Andrew, founder of an international ministry called Open Doors, has worked for decades in Muslim countries. He agrees that many Muslims see Jesus as Healer. He also prays for them in the name of Jesus (Isa).[36]

God's Other Powerful Names

Sometimes we focus so much on Jesus that we forget about God our Father (another person in the Trinity) and about the Lord our God (the full Trinity of Father, Son, and Spirit). We can also address those other names in our prayers.

Father God. Jesus taught His disciples to pray what we now call the Lord's Prayer. It begins: "… Our Father in heaven, hallowed be your name" (Matthew 6:9). One synonym for "hallowed" is "glorified." Glorified be the *name* of the Father.

In His prayer to the Father just before He was crucified, Jesus said: "I have manifested your name to the people whom you gave me out of the world" (John 17:6a). If Jesus wanted to manifest the name of the Father, so should we.

Lord God. The apostle James wrote:

> *Is anyone among you sick? Let him call for the elders of the church, and let them pray over him, anointing him with oil in the name of the Lord. And the prayer of faith will save the one who is sick, and the Lord will raise him up.*
>
> James 5:14–15a

Malachi 4:2 states: "…for you who fear my [the Lord's] name, the sun of righteousness shall rise with healing in its wings. You shall go out leaping like calves from the stall."

Proverbs 18:10 asserts: "The name of the Lord is a strong tower; the righteous man runs into it and is safe."

I also invite you to remember one of the Lord's covenant names, Jehovah Rapha (the Lord our Healer), revealed in Exodus 15:26.

Simply Call

In your toughest hours, you might not have the strength to pray long prayers. I encourage you to at least summon the strength to ask for healing and to then simply call out "Lord, Lord," or "Father, my Father," or "Jesus, Jesus."

Close your eyes and see those names written on the backdrop of your mind. Focus on them in your hour of need and find healing released by their limitless, timeless power.

Be healed, in the name of our Lord, in the name of Jehovah Rapha, in the name of our heavenly Father, and in the name of Jesus.

18

Value the Cross

I have watched our kids endure pain on various occasions. Such moments have been heart wrenching, particularly when, as a parent, I have authorized a painful medical procedure. One such time, I cried out to God, asking Him why He would allow my child to go through such severe pain. After I poured out my anguish, Father God quieted my soul. I sensed that He empathized with me as a parent, agonizing over my child's suffering. He reminded me that He had endured the pain of watching His Son go through something immeasurably worse. Father God had not just authorized a medical procedure; He had authorized His Son's death warrant.

My own pain that day subsided as I spent time thinking about what Jesus had endured before and during His crucifixion: the brutal crown of sharp thorns, the flesh-ripping and blood-splattering whippings, the struggle to carry the heavy cross, the pounding of huge nails into hands and feet, more blood pouring down, unquenchable thirst, the torture of a slow death—not to mention the incomprehensible pain of bearing all the sins, sorrows, and infirmities of the human race. Father God must have felt great anguish as He watched the crucifixion unfold. What is our human pain and suffering compared to that of Jesus and His Father that long-ago Friday in Jerusalem? That pain and suffering (and Father God's authorization of it) seem senseless until we come to fully understand the purpose of the cross.

Why Did Jesus Die?

Most importantly, Jesus died on the cross to save us from our spiritual sickness. He bore the sins of each one of us, taking up our punishment, giving up His own life as a sacrifice that was pleasing to Father God. Jesus made a way for us to enter into an everlasting relationship with God.

As a secondary matter (although still very important to you and me), Jesus bore our physical sicknesses and our infirmities on the cross. I know that there's debate in Christian circles about that secondary aspect of the cross. If you're among those who question that dual purpose for the cross, I invite you to consider the following verses.

Isaiah 53:5 states: "…he [Jesus] was pierced for our transgressions; he was crushed for our iniquities; upon him was the chastisement that brought us peace, and with his wounds we are healed."

Affirming that final phrase penned by the prophet Isaiah, the apostle Peter simply asserted: "By his [Jesus'] wounds you have been healed" (1 Peter 2:24b).

Not just saved. Healed. Both biblical passages talk about Jesus being wounded for us. Both passages claim that His wounds heal us.

The "wounds" referred to in Isaiah 53:5 were the marks on His body caused by the whipping Jesus received before He was crucified (Mark 15:15, Luke 22:63, John 19:1). In that era, Roman soldiers routinely flogged criminals before they crucified them, using whips with wooden handles that had several leather strips attached. Small iron balls or hooks, glass fragments, and sharp pieces of sheep bone were knotted at intervals into the leather strips. Such a torturous whip would have lashed many times across the bare back and legs of Jesus. The iron balls would have painfully bruised Him. The hooks, glass, and bone would have torn strips of flesh from His body, leaving stripes of bleeding muscle. No small matter, those wounds.

The NLT translation of Isaiah 53:5 reads: "… he was pierced for our rebellion, crushed for our sins. He was beaten so we could be whole. He was whipped so we could be healed."

Whatever the translation of the Isaiah 53 passage, the wording seems clear to me that Jesus suffered and then died for our sins *and* for our healing.

In his gospel, Matthew stated: "… [Jesus]… healed all who were sick. This was to fulfill what was spoken by the prophet Isaiah: 'He took our illnesses and bore our diseases'" (Matthew 8:16–17).

Matthew 8:17 proclaims and clarifies that the healing mentioned in Isaiah 53:5 refers to healing of our bodies, not just healing of our sin-strained relationship with God. (I dare to further submit that the words "illnesses" and "diseases" are broad enough to include mental and emotional illnesses as well.)

Many modern churches teach that Jesus died solely for the salvation of our sins. Thankfully, other churches teach that He died for the salvation *and* the healing of each one of us as *whole* persons. You have to decide which teaching you will believe.

Let's address this important issue from some further angles.

Jesus Showed He Cared about the Whole Person

It's not a stretch for me to believe that Jesus died for the healing of our spirits, our bodies, and our souls. While here on earth, Jesus didn't just treat people as spirits trapped in bodies of worthless clay. He cared about *every* aspect of each person: their spiritual state, their health, their mind, their emotions, and their relationships. He cared about the poor, the marginalized, and the outcasts. He helped and healed the sick, hurting, tormented, afflicted, and downtrodden people who came to Him. A fair review of all of His words and actions reveals that He cared about much more than the sin of humankind. He cared about the full range of human need.

Jesus sometimes healed people on the Sabbath, sending the message that He was as concerned about the restoration of the body as He was about the spirit's reformation.

I believe that He cared about our full selves right up until His final breath, and that His death on the cross provided the way for our *whole* beings to be reconciled with God. The cross forms the intersection of both the sin *and* the suffering of humanity with the love of God. When we enter into right standing with God, by accepting what Jesus did on the cross for us, we can be forgiven of our sins *and* we can ask God to heal us.

Our Bodies Are Worth Much

In 1 Corinthians 6:20, we learn from Paul that our *bodies* were bought with a great price (i.e. the death of Jesus on the cross). That's one reason God expects us to honour Him with our bodies. That verse offers further proof that Jesus didn't just die for our spiritual salvation; He died for us as whole beings, including our bodies.

The Greek Word *Sozo*

Paul, Luke, and others wrote a large portion of the New Testament in the Greek language (the main language spoken in the eastern Mediterranean world in their time). The Greek word *sozo* connotes both salvation *and* healing. [37]

In Romans 10:9, the word *sozo* is usually translated as "saved." That verse refers to a person being saved if they confess with their mouth that Jesus is Lord and believe in their heart that God has raised Jesus from the dead. In Acts 14:9, which deals with the physical healing of the man who was lame from birth, *sozo* is usually translated as "healed."

The use of the same word, *sozo*, to connote both salvation and healing further supports the argument that Jesus died for our whole selves (body, spirit, and soul).

The Concept of Atonement

In the Old Testament, the priests didn't just offer sacrifices to atone for the sins of the people. The priests used sacrifices to atone for physical impurities, as well. In Leviticus 14:18, for example, we learn that priests could atone for the cleansing of lepers. When Jesus died on the cross as the ultimate sacrifice, was it not for our *full* atonement? Dare we limit the atonement of Christ to our spirits only? Dare we make it less than the atonement human priests could offer in their acts of sacrifice? Why do so many churches today minister only to the spirit when parishioners also suffer in their bodies and souls, and Christ's atonement can cover it all?

The Curse Removed

The apostle Paul wrote: "Christ redeemed us from the curse of the law by becoming a curse for us, for it is written: 'Cursed is everyone who is hung on a pole'" (Galatians 3:13, NIV). Paul was, of course, referring to Christ hanging on the cross.

The curse of the law is described in detail in Deuteronomy 28. You can read that whole chapter for yourself, and you will see that the curse, arising from humankind's sin, included physical disease. When He hung on the cross, Jesus removed the whole curse of the law from us, including the curse of physical disease.

The Bread and the Wine

To remember what Jesus accomplished on the cross, we can participate in a practice called Communion (also known as the Lord's Supper or the Eucharist sacrament). If we belong to a community of believers, we can share in the regular observance of this deeply meaningful tradition. The apostle Paul taught about the practice of Communion in 1 Corinthians 11:17–34. In that passage, we learn that the bread we consume signifies Christ's broken body, and the wine we drink signifies His shed blood, reminding us of what He did for us on the cross (1 Corinthians 11:23–26).

According to Dr. Richard Swenson, who is both a scientist and a medical doctor, a few *drops* of human blood contain *billions* of red blood cells. We cannot calculate exactly how much blood Jesus shed on the cross, but from biblical descriptions of His crucifixion, we can safely assume that He lost more than a few drops of blood. Even if He lost *only* a few drops, Dr. Swenson has estimated that Jesus likely shed at least one red blood cell for every person who has ever lived. That means that at least one of His red blood cells had your name written on it.[38] I invite you to remember that thought the next time you participate in Communion.

Communion is a sacred ceremony. It must be respected, not treated lightly. The bread and the wine represent the most important event in the history of the world. We should not take Communion while we are still cherishing known sin that we have not yet confessed and turned away from. We should also abstain from Communion if we're not in a right relationship with our fellow Christians (insofar as that is within our control).

When the Corinthian church met together, the people "were not really interested in the Lord's Supper" (1 Corinthians 11:20, NLT). Some started eating the bread and drinking the wine without waiting for the others; some got drunk; others went hungry (vv. 21–22). This was partly because of divisions in the church. Paul warned them:

> ... *anyone who eats this bread or drinks this cup of the Lord*
> *unworthily is guilty of sinning against the body and blood of the*
> *Lord. That is why you should examine yourself before eating the*
> *bread and drinking the cup [and repent of unworthy behaviour*
> *towards God or man]. For if you eat the bread or drink the cup*
> *without honouring the body of Christ, you are eating and drinking*
> *God's judgment upon yourself. That is why many of you are*

weak and sick and some have even died. But if we would examine
ourselves, we would not be judged by God in this way.

1 Corinthians 11:27–31, NLT

According to Paul, taking Communion inappropriately and dishonourably can invite harm into our lives instead of the healing for which Jesus was whipped and wounded.

What if we instead choose to honour Christ's broken body and shed blood? Taking Communion in right standing with God and our fellow Christians invites the wounds of Jesus to generate the healing proclaimed by Isaiah 53:5 and 1 Peter 2:24.

The Full Power of the Cross

Ministries that offer both the salvation message and prayer for healing often draw large crowds and yield fantastic results in the realm of both body and spirit. Such combined ministries seem to be more prevalent in Latin America and Africa than in North America, which might explain the astonishing growth of evangelical and charismatic churches in those continents in recent decades.

This brings to mind the fascinating ministry of evangelist Reinhard Bonnke. Bonnke's ministry, Christ for all Nations, claims that since the 1970s, more than 70 million people have filled out decision cards indicating that they have positively responded to Bonnke's salvation invitation. Bonnke has held his outreaches in about fifty nations, including thirty-four African nations. He has a special love for Africa and draws enormous crowds there. At one single meeting in Lagos, Nigeria, in the year 2000, Bonnke preached to 1.6 million people, and about 1.1 million indicated they had accepted Christ during that meeting.

Bonnke usually preaches the same sermon: the basic good news of the gospel. He primarily focuses on the message of salvation, but Bonnke also prays for the sick. Bonnke presents Jesus as one who died for the whole person and who now, as the risen Son of God, still cares about each one of us on every level of our being.

Reports abound of the blind, deaf, and lame being healed at Bonnke's events. The crowds have grown exponentially over the years for reasons, including the stories of dramatic healings. Many Muslims have come to Christ because they have been healed.[39]

The message of Bonnke is clear: We can be saved from our sins because of the cross, but we can also be healed of our infirmities and diseases. The cross covers it all. I encourage you to find someone who preaches that Jesus died for us as whole beings.

Embrace the Full Power of the Cross

I don't want to cheapen or waste even one moment of the suffering of Jesus in His last hours, or even one drop of the blood that Jesus shed while on the cross. If I only accept forgiveness for my sins, then I'm not fully availing myself of all that His suffering and death were meant to accomplish. I want my sins forgiven *and* I want to be healed. I believe that I have been offered both forgiveness and healing by the finished work of Jesus on the cross. I want to fully receive all that has been revealed in Isaiah 53:4–5, 1 Peter 2:24, and Matthew 8:16–17.

Jesus cared so much about healing the sick and the suffering before He died. I believe He still cares about healing now. I choose to embrace the full power of the cross. Will you join me?

19

SEEK THE SPIRIT

Sitting beside the hospital beds of loved ones, I've found it sooth-ing to watch intravenous infusions dripping down through clear plastic tubing into their sick bodies. IV fluids contain much-needed hydration, nutrition, medication, and/or pain relief. The fluids con-tain a certain measure of healing power. Medically speaking, they can sometimes be all that separates life from death.

While praying, I've imagined the Holy Spirit flowing within the body of a sick person as a divine infusion. Jesus described the Spirit as a river of living water that can flow within us (John 7:38). Why settle for only medically administered IV fluids when we can also have the *living water* of the Spirit flowing through every nook and cranny of our bodies? The Spirit has more power, to an infinite degree, than any IV fluid, even chemotherapy.

The Spirit dwells in our bodies after we accept Christ into our lives (1 Corinthians 6:19). Pause to consider the enormity of that. Where the Spirit of the Lord is, there is *life*. We can welcome the Holy Spirit into every cell of our bodies. We can imagine His living water flowing within. The Holy Spirit can refresh us, revive us, and restore us.

Ezekiel 47:9c describes a river of healing: "Life will flourish wher-ever this water flows" (NLT). Some commentators suggest that this river signifies the Spirit's healing water flowing within believers (like the river Jesus described).

We should value the blessed wonders of modern medicine, but sooner or later, we all realize that medical science does not provide a cure for all health problems. Thankfully, the Spirit's power extends beyond the limitations of science. Accept IV fluids, of course, but also accept the divine infusion of the Spirit that God offers.

Romans 8:11 reveals this marvellous truth: The same Spirit that raised Christ from the dead dwells in us! If the Spirit can overcome death, surely the Spirit can overcome cancer, or heart disease, or anything else that ails us. The Spirit can trickle within us like a stream diminished by drought or flow like a mighty river in the season of rain. This depends, to some extent, on how much we receive or resist the Spirit from day to day. It also depends on us clearing sin out of our lives. Sin will obstruct or diminish the river of living water. Once known sin is dealt with, we can invite more of the Spirit to come into our lives by drawing close to God and His people, meditating on God's words, and praying.

Does your church teach much about the Holy Spirit? Some churches focus primarily on Jesus. Yet the Spirit is also an important member of the Trinity. The Bible contains many references to the Holy Spirit. I encourage you to get to know Him.

I wish had the space to discuss references to the Spirit in the Old Testament. You can discover for yourself references that begin as early as Genesis 1:2, which declares that the Spirit hovered over the earth and its waters at creation. You can read about how the Spirit came upon Moses, Joshua, Samson, David, and Isaiah for limited periods of time.

The Spirit is mentioned often in the New Testament. Jesus received the Holy Spirit after He was baptized. The heavens opened up and the Spirit descended on Him (Luke 3:22). After this, Jesus began performing miracles.

Jesus relied on the power of the Spirit to heal people who came to Him. We're told in Acts 10:37–38: "You know... how God anointed

Jesus of Nazareth with the Holy Spirit and power, and how he went around doing good and healing... because God was with him" (NIV).

Jesus promised that the gift of the Spirit would come to His apostles *and* to all those who would believe in Him through them (John 17:20). Jesus didn't just leave His followers with words. He left earth pledging to them a measure of His power. We cannot live our Christians lives to their full potential without that power.

After He died, Jesus appeared on earth over a period of forty days, further teaching His apostles:

> *And while staying with them he [Jesus] ordered them not to depart from Jerusalem, but to wait for the promise of the Father, which, he [Jesus] said, "you heard from me; for John baptized with water, but you will be baptized with the Holy Spirit not many days from now... you will receive power when the Holy Spirit has come upon you ..."*
>
> Acts 1:4–5, 8

Similar words of Jesus were recorded at Luke 24:49: "And behold, I am sending the promise of my Father upon you. But stay in the city [Jerusalem] until you are clothed with power from on high."

After Jesus ascended from this world, the apostles obediently gathered together in Jerusalem. On the day of Pentecost:

> *... suddenly there came from heaven a sound like a mighty rushing wind, and it filled the entire house where they were sitting. And divided tongues as of fire appeared to them and rested on each one of them. And they were all filled with the Holy Spirit...*
>
> Acts 2:2–4

From that point on, those men had the power of God flowing in them and through them. They didn't just *talk* about God the Father and Jesus the Son in the years that followed. They accessed and demonstrated God's mighty power.

Seek the Spirit   191

We've already briefly considered the Acts 3 story of a destitute man who had been crippled for forty years. The man asked Peter and John for money as they approached the Temple, a few days after Pentecost. Peter told the man: "I have no silver and gold, but what I do have I give to you. In the name of Jesus Christ of Nazareth, rise up and walk" (v. 6). Peter extended his right hand and helped the lame man to his feet. The man began to leap around.

This amazed people and alarmed the Jewish authorities. The religious leaders detained Peter and John and tried to intimidate them into promising that they would stop speaking and teaching in the name of Jesus. The city was still abuzz about the crucifixion of Jesus and there was already much talk of Jesus having appeared to many people in resurrected form. Peter and John refused to agree to stop talking in the name of Jesus, "for we cannot but speak about what we have seen and heard" (Acts 4:20).

After being released, Peter and John visited their fellow believers, who prayed with the two apostles:

And now, Lord, look upon their [the religious elders'] threats and grant to your servants to continue to speak your word with all boldness, while you stretch out your hand to heal, and signs and wonders are performed through the name of your holy servant Jesus.

Acts 4:29–30

I love what happened after that. Acts 4:31 reveals: "And when they had prayed, the place in which they were gathered together was shaken, and they were all filled with the Holy Spirit and continued to speak the word of God with boldness."

After being filled afresh with a measure of the Spirit, "... many signs and wonders were regularly done among the people by the hands of the apostles" (Acts 5:12a). Those signs and wonders included healing.

When Peter walked through crowds in Jerusalem, he had ongoing power to heal. Peter was so full of the indwelling Spirit that his simple presence caused healing:

... more and more men and women believed in the Lord and were
added to their number [the number of believers]. As a result,
people brought the sick into the streets and laid them on beds and
mats so that at least Peter's shadow might fall on some of them
as he passed by. Crowds also gathered from the towns around
Jerusalem, bringing their sick and those tormented by evil spirits,
and all of them were healed.

Acts 5:14–16, NIV

Can you imagine the *shadow* of Peter being full of healing power? We've talked about the shadow of death (Psalm 23:4). In contrast, Peter's shadow was full of life.

The Spirit also moved mightily through the apostle Paul. Throughout this book, you'll read stories of how God used Paul to heal many. In Acts 19:11–12, we're told: "God did extraordinary miracles through Paul, so that even handkerchiefs and aprons that had touched him were taken to the sick, and their illnesses were cured..." (NIV)

Paul wrote to the Christians in Corinth:

And I was with you in weakness and in fear and much trem-
bling, and my speech and my message were not in plausible
words of wisdom, but in demonstration of the Spirit and of
power, so that your faith might not rest in the wisdom of men but
in the power of God.

1 Corinthians 2:3–5

Paul wrote to ordinary believers in Galatia that *they* could, by faith, receive "the promised Holy Spirit" (Galatians 3:14, NLT).

In Acts 8:6–7, we read about how the Spirit moved through Philip: "When the crowds heard Philip and saw the signs he performed, they all paid close attention to what he said... and many who were paralyzed or lame were healed" (NIV).

If you want to read more about how the disciples, apostles, and many others were filled with the Spirit, and thereafter demonstrated

God's power, I encourage you to read the whole book of Acts. It has twenty-eight chapters. If you read a chapter a day, you can finish that New Testament book in four weeks. Acts describes God's love and power *in action* as the Spirit moved within and around the early Christians. I believe that the book of Acts is a model for dynamic, present-day Christian living, not just a history lesson.

Are you one of those who think that God granted the Spirit only to the apostles? Do you believe that such an astonishing gift was only available for a limited time for a limited few? If so, I invite you to consider what Peter told the crowds after the apostles were filled with the Spirit on the day of Pentecost:

> *... Repent and be baptized every one of you in the name of Jesus Christ for the forgiveness of your sins, and you will receive the gift of the Holy Spirit. For the promise is for you and for all your children and for all who are far off, everyone whom the Lord our God calls to himself.*
>
> Acts 2:38–39

You. All your children. All who were/are far off, in time and space, from the moment those words were spoken. Every believer.

Has the Holy Spirit grown old and tired? Has He lost His power? Does God no longer want His Spirit to indwell and empower believers in *our* age? Does He want today's believers to be weak and powerless? The potent forces of evil, darkness, and disease are still clearly alive and well, and they come against believers. Why would God refuse to grant the overcoming power of His Spirit to His people in *this* age? I will go on the record as one who believes that the same Spirit that raised Christ from the dead is alive in *us* (Romans 8:11). I pray that every reader fully comprehends the truth and reality of that verse.

In *this* hour, God doesn't just give us wise words to live by. He offers us the Spirit's power, to live as we ought, to help and bless others. God wants to demonstrate His power in many ways, including healing the sick through believers willing to yield to the Spirit's flow of living water.

A Special Measure of the Spirit's Power

Paul taught the early church that each person could receive special gifts from the Spirit, including enhanced gifts of knowledge, healing, and miraculous powers. He wrote to the church at Corinth:

> *Now concerning spiritual gifts, brothers, I do not want you to be uninformed... Now there are varieties of gifts, but the same Spirit; and there are varieties of service, but the same Lord; and there are varieties of activities, but it is the same God who empowers them all in everyone. To each is given the manifestation of the Spirit for the common good. For to one is given through the Spirit the utterance of wisdom, and to another the utterance of knowledge according to the same Spirit, to another faith by the same Spirit, to another gifts of healing by the one Spirit, to another the working of miracles... All these are empowered by one and the same Spirit, who apportions to each one individually as he wills.*
>
> 1 Corinthians 12:1, 4–11

The apostle Paul compared the Body of Christ (all those who believe) to the human body, which consists of feet, hands, ears, eyes, a nose, and other parts. All have their own particular function. They work together in harmony and bless the body as a whole. The church also has many individual parts, and each one has their own function. Each one contributes to the wellbeing of the whole.

Miracles and gifts of healing are again referred to in 1 Corinthians 12:28–30: "And God has appointed in the church first apostles, second prophets, third teachers, then miracles, then gifts of healing... Do all work miracles? Do all possess gifts of healing?" Paul didn't directly answer those questions, but the passage as a whole implies that only some people receive the specified gifts.

Paul instructed Christians to "earnestly desire the higher gifts" (1 Corinthians 12:31). The gifts of healing and working miracles are in the middle of the list (not the highest gifts, but also not the most common).

The Spirit can anoint a person with the gift of healing. This gift allows a *special* augmented measure of God's power to flow through them as they pray over a person. They can pray with heightened faith and authority, sensing that the Spirit is empowering them in an exceptional way. The gift of healing is sometimes accompanied by the gift of knowledge. Perhaps the person so gifted will receive some specific knowledge about the person(s) they are praying for (that they would not otherwise have known), such as some detail about their physical ailment. The gift of healing might also be accompanied by the gift of faith (an unusual measure of faith) and/or the gift of working miracles.

The gift of healing is not granted permanently to anyone but is given at particular moments for the healing of one or more people. When the gift is in operation, the person being prayed for may be healed immediately, in whole, or in part.

We can ask God for the gift of healing to be bestowed upon us by the Spirit before we pray for someone's healing. We should not *presume* to have the gift. We will *know* when the Spirit is giving that extra measure of power to us as we pray.

I believe that I have been in the presence of people with the gift of healing on a few occasions. On one occasion, for example, a pastor I didn't know prayed for a family member. The pastor prayed specifically for the healing of this person's bones, even though he hadn't been asked to do so, even though he had no idea what their medical status was or that the person had been taking high doses of a drug that can weaken bones. I believe that this pastor had been given special revelation of the medical situation. This person's bones were shown to be amazingly healthy on a bone scan that was later done—quite a miracle in light of the steroid doses that had been taken over many years.

We must not confuse the special gift of healing with the everyday ability of each one of us to pray for healing. We can pray for healing at any time. If we have right standing with God, the Spirit is *always* present within us in *some* measure. It's up to the Spirit to decide whether to do something extraordinary in the moment. Prayer can still be powerful without the special gifts of healing, knowledge, or miracle working in operation. The operation of the gifts can create an added boost of power, but such gifts aren't always present, or necessary, when we pray for healing.

The Everyday Presence of the Spirit

I will repeat this essential point: *Any* authentic believer has a measure of the Spirit within them and can pray with faith for the healing of themselves and others. We can ask the indwelling Spirit to flow through every cell of our bodies when we're sick, and we can ask for Him to flow through us to others struggling with health issues.

We can ask the Spirit for more than healing. The Spirit has further roles, such as being our comforter (John 14:26) and our constant companion. The Spirit can provide a divine measure of peace, calm, faith, assurance, strength, hope, and encouragement. In a time of sickness and suffering, we often need much more than physical healing, especially if the healing doesn't come right away. The apostle Paul told us that we are to "live by the Spirit" (Galatians 5:5, NLT). We can ask God to freshly fill us with the Spirit each day.

We can ask the Spirit to intercede for us. Romans 8:26 advises that when we don't know exactly what to pray, the Spirit will act as our intercessor, praying to Father God on our behalf. The Spirit is our most valuable intercessor. When we're too weak, tired, and sick to pray, we can ask the Spirit to pray for us with all the perfect pleas He knows. What a precious privilege!

I encourage you to seek more of the Spirit's presence, to ask for a greater flow of living water within. The Spirit is full of God's healing power and so much more!

20

STEP OUT WITH AUTHORITY

Before Jesus died, He transferred some of His healing *authority* to others. Matthew 10:1 reveals: "... he called to him his twelve disciples and gave them authority... to heal every disease and every affliction."

Luke also described that transfer of authority: "And he [Jesus] called the twelve together and gave them power and authority... to cure diseases, and he sent them out to proclaim the kingdom of God and to heal" (Luke 9:1–2).

The transfer of authority was effective. Luke recorded: "And they [the twelve] departed and went through the villages, preaching the gospel and healing everywhere" (Luke 9:6).

Jesus then gave others (beyond the twelve) the authority to heal:

After this the Lord appointed seventy-two others and sent them
on ahead of him, two by two, into every town and place where he
himself was about to go... [instructing them:] Heal the sick... and
say to them, "The kingdom of God has come near to you."

Luke 10:1, 9

When the seventy-two returned to Him, elated at what had happened on their journeys, Jesus said to them: "Behold, I have given you authority to tread on serpents and scorpions, and over all the power of the enemy…" (Luke 10:19). Is sickness our friend or our enemy? I hope you agree with me that sickness is our enemy.

After His ascension, Jesus sent the Spirit to His followers, as we discussed in the last chapter. Believers then had even greater power and authority in the realm of healing. The Spirit no longer temporarily empowered believers. He came to *dwell* within each believer in some measure.

The transfer of power and authority from Jesus to us today can be traced back to words Jesus said before His crucifixion:

> *Truly, truly, I say to you, whoever believes in me will also do the*
> *works that I do; and greater works than these will he do, because*
> *I am going to the Father. Whatever you ask in my name, this I*
> *will do, that the Father may be glorified in the Son. If you ask me*
> *anything in my name, I will do it.*
>
> John 14:12–14

Jesus wasn't just talking to His disciples about what *they* could do after He was gone. Jesus said that "whoever believes in me" would be able to do even greater works than Him. *Whoever*. That's a broad enough word to include you and me.

Just as Jesus sent out the twelve, the seventy-two, and then further believers, He still sends out believers today, equipping them with His power and authority to heal.

Has the modern church forgotten what Jesus said about believers being able to do even greater works than Him? Yes, in part.

Let's add to the brief look we've already taken at church history over the two millennia since Jesus left this earth. Most of what I discuss below derives from two books written by Francis MacNutt, *Healing* and *The Healing Reawakening*.[40]

The early church taught that ordinary believers could be channels of God's power, imparting healing to the sick. Christian writers of that era, such as Justin Martyr, Irenaeus, Cyprian, and Tertullian, recorded that church history. Modern writers, such as Yale professor Dr. Ramsay MacMullen, opine that Christianity grew explosively throughout the Roman Empire in the first three centuries after Christ, mainly because Christians demonstrated they could access God's power to heal the sick.[41]

After those first three centuries, some theologians began to believe and teach that the age of healing had ceased. They arbitrarily put an expiry date on the words of Jesus recorded in John 14:12–13. Yet Jesus never said that His followers would only be able to perform greater works than Him for a few centuries.

In the fifth century, Augustine believed that healing authority was no longer available. He changed his opinion a few years before he died. He wrote in his book *Retractions* that he no longer believed that the age of miracles was over. He had seen too many people divinely healed in his lifetime. But by then, an increasing number of other theologians were adopting the view that the age of healing had passed. Theological focus shifted to the soul and spirit. Salvation was no longer offered for the whole person, but only for the inner self.

The belief that every Christian has authority to pray for healing became even further eroded after the fifth century. In the Catholic Church, the laity was told they could no longer pray for healing. Only priests and bishops could perform that prayer rite. Even clergy eventually stopped praying for healing for several centuries. The priestly sacrament of the Last Anointing (also known as the Extreme Unction) replaced the Anointing of the Sick. A priest would come to pray only when an ill person lay on their deathbed.

In some nations, and for many centuries, healing was only expected to occur in special Catholic shrines or because of the prayers of rare holy people who were worthy of sainthood. St. Ferrer and St. Catherine of Siena are examples of Catholic saints known for healing the sick in the fourteenth century.

Then, in some countries, royalty claimed a monopoly on healing. In England in the sixteenth century, King Henry VIII declared that only he had the power to pray for healing. Not even clergy were allowed to pray for their parishioners anymore. In the seventeenth century, King Charles I made it illegal for anyone other than the monarch to pray for healing.

Belief that ordinary Christians could pray for healing was pretty much gone by the sixteenth-century Protestant Reformation. One theologian of that era, John Calvin, began teaching the doctrine of cessationism, which held that supernatural healing through Christ's followers stopped after the last apostle died. Calvin's teachings have influenced many Protestant denominations right up to this present age (although some modern Calvinists have revived belief in the power of healing prayer).

And then came the Enlightenment in the eighteenth century. Intellectuals began to believe in science. Scientists became increasingly wary of religion, and they began to influence various Protestant denominations. Liberal Protestants began to question whether the healing miracles of Jesus actually happened.

During the Great Awakening of the eighteenth century, some Protestant clergy tried to reignite belief in healing prayer. Pockets of believers here and there tried to resurrect healing prayer, but there was substantial pushback by the church as an institution.

In the nineteenth century, John Nelson Darby developed the Theory of Dispensationalism, which taught that healing (and other gifts of the Spirit) occurred only in the apostolic era, in the first century after Christ, because of a unique dispensation. Darby influenced prominent Protestant Christians of his era, such as Dwight L. Moody and C. I. Scofield.

Along the way, theology also developed (in both Catholic and Protestant churches) that granted noble status to the state of suffering. (We will spend a later chapter talking about the many good things that can arise from suffering. Recognizing that suffering has a constructive side is different from making suffering a virtuous aspiration.) Many Christians began believing that because suffering was so important in the quest for holiness, it was wrong to pray for healing. Suffering was cherished as if it conferred an invisible halo.

In the early 1900s, a revival of belief in healing prayer developed in some denominations. It began most notably in Pentecostal churches. This movement has since spread into many churches. The Catholic Church now has a strong charismatic segment. The Anointing of the Sick sacrament has been officially restored. Many evangelical churches have rediscovered a vital belief in healing prayer. The modern healing movement across diverse denominations encourages ordinary people, not just priests or pastors, to pray for healing.

Do *you* believe in the statement Jesus made in John 14:12–13, that *whoever* believes in Him will be able to do the same (and even greater) works as He did? If so, begin (or keep on!) using the power and authority He has granted you. You can do great works if you step out in faith, believing in Him, praying for healing for yourself and others (because He said you can).

The Laying on of Hands

Jesus laid hands on the sick. Jairus must have seen Jesus do so, because he implored Jesus: "My little daughter is at the point of death. Come and lay your hands on her, so that she may be made well and live" (Mark 5:23). By the time Jesus arrived at the home of Jairus, the little girl was dead. Undeterred, Jesus took her by the hand and told her to rise up. Immediately, she got up and walked (Mark 5:41–42).

On other occasions: Jesus reached out with His hand and touched a leper who was then healed (Matthew 8:3, Mark 1:41–42); Jesus touched the hand of Peter's sick mother-in-law and her fever then left her (Matthew 8:15); and Jesus touched the eyes of blind men as He healed them (Matthew 9:29; 20:34).

In Luke 13:10–13, we read about a woman who had been bent over and crippled for eighteen years. When Jesus saw her, He declared: "Woman, you are freed from your disability" (v. 12). Then he laid His hands on her and "… immediately she was made straight, and she glorified God" (v. 13).

Jesus laid hands on many other sick people: "At sunset, the people brought to Jesus all who had various kinds of sickness, and laying his hands on each one, he healed them" (Luke 4:40, NIV).

Paul also laid his hands on the sick and they were healed:

His father [the father of the chief official of Malta] was sick in bed, suffering from fever and dysentery. Paul went in to see him and, after prayer, placed his hands on him and healed him. When this had happened, the rest of the sick on the island came and were cured.

Acts 28:8–9, NIV

I have read about an American evangelist in Argentina named Tommy Hicks. In 1954, he rented a stadium in Buenos Aires that seated 25,000 people and held a series of public meetings there. One day, a stadium guard told Hicks about his pain. Hicks laid hands on him and the man was instantly healed. Later, Hicks had the opportunity to meet Peron, the President of Argentina, who had a disfiguring skin disease. Hicks prayed for Peron while holding the President's hand. Peron's skin cleared. Word about what God was doing through Hicks spread. Crowds overflowed the first stadium. Hicks moved to a larger stadium that seated more than 100,000. About three million Argentinians attended Hicks' meetings over the next two months, and many were healed (although I don't suppose that Hicks could lay his hands on all of them).[42]

Mark 16:17–18 informs us that *we* can lay hands on the sick: "And these signs will accompany *those who believe*: in my name… they will lay their hands on the sick, and they will recover." All that's required of the person laying their hands on the sick is that they do so in the name of Jesus and that they believe in Him. The simple promise that Jesus made to believers in Mark 16:17–18 contains so much power! Have you ever deliberately laid your hands on a sick person (with their permission) as you prayed for them?

When we dare to lay hands on someone and pray for them, we don't always know the full range of their needs. But God knows, and

His power can flow through us. I love a story told by renowned Bible smuggler Brother Andrew about a man named George, who acted as Brother Andrew's interpreter in Cuba years ago. One evening, as Brother Andrew prepared to speak at a church in Havana, he noticed George praying. George, who suffered from a chronic digestive order, was silently asking God to take away his pain so he could focus on interpreting Brother Andrew's message. Not knowing why George was praying so intensely, Brother Andrew walked up behind him. He laid his hands on George's shoulders and prayed quietly for him. Much later, Brother Andrew learned that George's pain dissipated while Brother Andrew prayed. George became permanently free of the digestive disorder from that day onward.[43]

God can do wonderful things through the laying on of hands, even if our faith is somewhat ambivalent (perhaps because our feelings for the person being prayed for are complicated). I remember visiting a woman in the hospital some years ago who had said hurtful things to me in the past. As I stood at the woman's bedside, I saw how pain-wracked she was. God nudged me deep within. Sensing He wanted me to lay hands on this woman, I asked for her consent to do so. I felt an inner prompting to pray out loud for her healing. I didn't particularly want to, but I knew I had to. As I placed my hands on her and began to pray, compassion filled me that I *knew* originated from the Spirit, *not* from my own natural feelings at that time. I was surprised at the tender words that came out of my mouth.

After a few minutes, I felt a bright light shimmering behind my closed eyelids. I also felt an unusual sensation, like an electric current, flowing from my hands into the woman's body. An unmistakable power flowed through me. To this day, I marvel that God used *imperfect* me, full of conflicted feelings, to deliver His healing power to this woman. She fully recovered soon after.

Such is the power of obediently laying hands on the sick as we pray for them. We don't have to have a wellspring of good feelings for them to obey God's instruction. Patients in pain can often be irritable, maybe even rude. They can seem unappreciative of our effort to visit or our offer to pray. We don't have to have warm and fuzzy feelings for them at the moment we lay hands on them and pray. When we do lay hands on them, we won't necessarily feel power passing through our hands. We must simply trust that it is flowing. In my experience, it's rare to feel any warmth or surge.

It has been a special privilege to lay hands, without ambivalence, on dearly loved family members and close friends. The touch of genuine love is *always* full of spiritual voltage, whether we *feel* any powerful current moving through our hands or not.

I believe that we can also lay hands on our own bodies. When I was severely ill with C. *difficile*, I spoke aloud to my body and laid hands on myself. I commanded the harmful bacteria to be flushed out of my bowel in orderly fashion. I commanded all good bacteria in my gut to multiply. I asked the Spirit to move, through my hands laid on my abdomen, into my weakened body. Something about the act of laying my hands on my own body strengthened my faith and enabled my feeble body to get to the hospital. Recovery followed diagnosis and treatment.

Speaking with Authority

We can choose to speak against disease, disability, and dysfunction with words of authority. Let's dare to speak to cancer cells and command them to shrivel up and die. Let's forbid them from multiplying. Let's speak to healthy cells and tell them to multiply appropriately. I have seen that kind of prayer prayed effectively over people whose cancer has soon gone into remission for many years. We can speak with authority against *any* diseased or dysfunctional cells, against infection and inflammation, and against harmful viruses and bacteria.

God created the world with words. The first chapter of Genesis records how God *spoke* light, sky, land, oceans, vegetation, living creatures, and humankind into existence with words such as: "Let there be..."

Jesus used words to command disease or disability to leave individuals. He commanded eyes to see, ears to hear, tongues to speak, and lame legs to walk.

Jesus said that if we have faith, we can speak to a mountain and command it to move from here to there, or even to fall into the sea (Matthew 17:20; 21:21; Mark 11:23). Surely if we can command a mountain to tumble into the sea, we can command tiny cancer cells to be destroyed. Jesus told a fig tree to shrivel up and die, and it did, setting a precedent for commanding the destruction of living matter.

Do we have anything to lose by speaking words of authority? Maybe we'll appear foolish, putting ourselves at risk of ridicule or failure. Who cares? If Jesus told us to use our spoken words to command a situation to change, then we should obey Him and trust Him for the results. Will the results be instant? Not likely. We can *keep on* speaking words in faith, even after medical help is sought.

Words have the power of life and death (Proverbs 18:21). Even if you believe you're dealing with a terminal illness, you can declare: "I shall not die, but I shall live, and recount the deeds of the Lord" (Psalm 118:17).

Perhaps an ailing loved one lives far away. We can phone them, if possible. If not, we can speak a prayer out loud in the privacy of our home. I've come to trust that my words can travel to a sick person (not audibly, but in the spiritual realm). If manmade phone cables and satellites can carry our words thousands of kilometres away, can't the Spirit do the same thing for us in a dimension beyond our five senses? Although the sick person won't hear the words, the words can still have effect.

Anointing with Oil

James 5:14–15a states:

> *Is anyone among you sick? Let him call for the elders of the*
> *church, and let them pray over him, anointing him with oil in the*
> *name of the Lord. And the prayer of faith will save the one who is*
> *sick, and the Lord will raise him up.*

I encourage you to avail yourself of this course of action. I did so when I received my diagnosis of skin cancer. Sam was anointed with oil and prayed for by a pastor during his time in the ICU with a brain bleed. We've sought anointing with oil whenever we've battled serious health issues in our family.

Blessed oil represents the Holy Spirit. I'm hearing about many denominations restoring the practice of anointing the sick with oil while praying for their recovery. In 1974, the Catholic Church restored the "Anointing of the Sick" sacrament.[44] Priests are once again visiting ill parishioners before they're on their deathbeds. They are laying hands on them, praying, *and* anointing them with oil, fulfilling what James 5:14–16 prescribes.

Acting on Our Authority

I invite you to take up the power and authority that Jesus granted you. Seek out mature Christians and church elders who are willing to do the same. I pray that boldness, faith, and courage visibly mark His believers and His current church as noticeably as they long ago marked the early church. Let's see what God does in response.

21

Seek Medical Help

In my forties, I developed high blood pressure. This didn't surprise me, given my family history and stressful law career. I wasn't concerned at first, believing I could simply handle the problem through prayer.

Sometimes I used an inflatable cuff, offered to local pharmacy customers, to check my blood pressure. The numbers that popped up on the electronic screen dismayed me. I tried to fool the cuff. I purposely used it when I felt relaxed or on days when I reduced my caffeine intake. It didn't matter. The numbers remained bothersome.

I tried to further change my lifestyle. I walked more. I cut back on salt. I ate bananas and drank even less coffee. I learned more about stress management. Those wise strategies helped, to some extent, but I eventually realized that I couldn't realistically exercise every day. When eating out, I couldn't completely control the salt added to meals. And I couldn't bear giving up coffee entirely.

My doctor kept recommending that I go on blood pressure medication. She couldn't understand why I was so against the idea. She finally convinced me to wear a round-the-clock monitor. The results revealed that my average blood pressure was worse than I thought, even during the night. Changes in lifestyle were clearly not working as well as I'd hoped. Prayer had probably prevented a heart attack or stroke, but it hadn't fully solved the situation. I finally relented. In my early fifties, I went on blood pressure medication.

The first medication that my doctor prescribed made me cough almost incessantly. She switched me to another pill. Thankfully, it had no discernable side effects. It brought my blood pressure down to the normal range. I no longer dreaded inflating the cuff.

I began to thank God for providing the miracle pill I take every morning. Medication became my friend. God used my doctor's advice and the medication she prescribed to answer years of prayer. (Of course, I still walk, use salt and caffeine in moderation, and try to manage stress, because those efforts matter too.)

My story is not unusual. Many Christians believe that they should rely primarily on God and their own efforts when dealing with health issues. Francis MacNutt has written about the "artificial opposition" some Christians create between their Christian faith and medicine.[45]

God has blessed us with doctors, other health professionals, surgical options, and medication. We should not lightly reject any of these wonderful resources *if* they are available. Seeking medical treatment does not negate faith. In many cases, it takes *great* faith to undergo a medical procedure, such as major surgery, or to use medication with lots of potential side effects. Some loved ones have undergone surgery or taken medications after being bluntly told that death was a potential risk.

I think of a friend named Jim who was diagnosed with stage-four kidney cancer in his early seventies. The cancer had already metastasized in his lungs, spleen, and some bones. After meeting with a top oncologist who specialized in kidney surgeries, Jim agreed to the removal of the diseased kidney. The doctor warned that the surgery would be complicated because malignant tissue from one of the tumours lodged on that kidney had wrapped itself around the nearby vena cava vein (one of the largest blood vessels in the body). The surgeon frankly told my friend that there was a high probability he wouldn't survive the surgery. If the vena cava vein was nicked, Jim could bleed to death on the operating table. The surgeon advised my friend to get his affairs in order before the operation. Can you imagine the off-the-charts faith it took to sign the surgery consent form? Jim took courage in a verse God had highlighted in his spirit. Thankfully, Jim survived the surgery. God gave him several further months with his family and friends.

I strongly encourage you to consider adding medical means to the spiritual resources we've discussed. God can, and often does, use medical help to extend our lives.

If you're making medical decisions for others, such as your children, you might have a legal obligation to seek medical help (depending on the circumstances and what jurisdiction you live in). I read about a Wisconsin couple sentenced to 180 days in jail because their eleven-year-old daughter died of untreated diabetes in 2009. The couple had decided *not* to seek medical help but to rely only on prayer. That same year, a couple in Pennsylvania was charged with involuntary manslaughter after their two-year-old son died from untreated bacterial pneumonia.[46] Caregivers need to be wise and responsible. They should not foolishly resist available medical treatment.

Medical Professionals

I hope you live in a community where you can seek the help of doctors and other kinds of medical professionals. Highly educated, they have much to offer. I've benefitted from many experienced, caring, diligent medical professionals. I've found it a huge relief to hand a health concern over to them (after also handing it over to God). Their advice and treatment have helped to resolve many health issues.

My husband has practised medicine for almost four decades. You can imagine the expertise he has developed. Countless patients have told me how much he has helped them. In some cases, God has used Sam to save lives.

Jesus mentioned a medical doctor in a conversation with religious leaders (who were upset that Jesus had dined with a house full of sinners). After hearing their criticism, Jesus said: "Healthy people don't need a doctor—sick people do" (Matthew 9:12b, NLT). Although Jesus was speaking about *spiritual* health, His use of the doctor metaphor showed respect. He was, in effect, referring to Himself as a doctor (which has given rise to a nickname, the Great Physician). His regard for the medical profession contrasts with the disdain He held for self-righteous religious leaders.

Although I firmly believe that it's wise to get medical help when warranted, we should not rely *exclusively* on human help. Our ultimate reliance must remain on God, our Creator and sustainer. Consider this story about King Asa (Solomon's great grandson):

> *In the thirty-ninth year of his reign [King] Asa was diseased in his feet, and his disease became severe. Yet even in his disease he did not seek the Lord, but sought help from the physicians. And Asa slept with his fathers, dying in the forty-first year of his reign.*
>
> 2 Chronicles 16:12–13

King Asa probably had severe gout, a condition that would have caused him to limp around in agony. I don't think God was displeased that King Asa sought medical help. I believe that God allowed King Asa's disease to increase in severity until his death because the king had not simultaneously sought God's help.

Doctors, even in our day, have vast but limited knowledge. They can help us a lot, but they cannot heal everyone of everything. Modern medicine hasn't fully conquered heart disease, or all forms of cancer, or many other diseases. Only God has unlimited power to heal. God's healing power outweighs humanity's medical power by an incalculable degree.

The Bible tells a story about a woman with a bleeding disorder who had consulted many doctors: "… there was a woman who had a discharge of blood for twelve years, and who had suffered much under many physicians, and had spent all that she had, and was no better but rather grew worse" (Mark 5:25–26).

I don't think this passage criticizes the woman for consulting doctors. It simply reveals that doctors are not God. Even going to the most renowned doctors, or seeking the most expensive medical therapy, doesn't guarantee healing. All the money in the world cannot buy health and healing. I thank God that when we reach the limits of what human medicine can offer, He still reigns in heaven and can reach down to help us. Jesus healed the woman with the bleeding disorder. God can heal what doctors cannot. Seeking God's help shouldn't rule out the help of medical professionals. Conversely, seeking medical help should not sideline God's help.

God honours our efforts to keep Him in the picture even when we have access to the best of medical help. In 2013, a friend in her mid-thirties, who was living far from her home country, developed a growth on her eyelid in a short period of time. She looked back at photographs of her face from just months before, and the strange mole was not there. A doctor friend in her home country said that she should get it checked out because it seemed unusual. Concerned, my friend went to her doctor in the foreign location where she was living. The doctor suspected melanoma because of the colour, appearance, and rapid growth of the eyelid mole. Melanoma, which can be deadly, is the most serious form of skin cancer.

My friend prayed about the situation, asking God to help her connect with the right specialist to confirm the diagnosis and perform surgery. My friend was concerned that surgery on her eyelid would be disfiguring, because the surgeon would likely cut a margin of healthy tissue around the growth to make sure he got all of the suspected cancer cells. She was also somewhat anxious that such a delicate surgery would take place in a foreign country by a surgeon she didn't know, even though he practised in a reputable facility.

I encouraged her to see a surgeon but also suggested that she concurrently pray for divine healing. Sometimes when the need is urgent, we get so busy seeking out medical help that we don't pause to ask God for His superlative healing power to come down. God could do far and beyond what even the best medical specialist in the world could do. My friend agreed with my suggestion and began to pray for divine healing.

She still proceeded to consult a plastic surgeon, who set a date for surgery. Before her scheduled surgery, God healed her. The growth began to shrink and then it disappeared without any medical intervention. Both my friend and the surgeon were quite surprised. Although tentative about attributing the outcome to God, my friend recognized that the outcome seemed somewhat miraculous. She told the surgeon that she believed she had been divinely healed. He couldn't refute her. What other explanation could there be?

Sometimes we *do* need to undergo surgery. My point remains simply this: While we put one foot in front of the other in the medical system, we can *also* pray for God to heal us and give Him due credit when the healing comes.

One modern symbol of medical healing is a serpent winding itself around a pole. There's both a biblical and a mythological history to that symbol. The biblical narrative (Numbers 21:1–9) begins with Moses leading the Israelites to the Promised Land after their deliverance from slavery in Egypt. As they wandered in the wilderness, the impatient Israelites "spoke against God and Moses" (v. 5). "Then the Lord sent fiery serpents among the people, and they bit the people, so that many people of Israel died" (v. 6). The people confessed their sin then beseeched Moses to pray that the Lord would take away the serpents. After Moses prayed, God told him to make a bronze serpent and place it on a pole. Anyone who looked at the pole after being bitten by a snake would live. Moses obediently made a snake-entwined pole. Those who gazed at it survived poisonous snakebites. The pole became an instrument and a symbol of healing and life.

Then the Israelites began to worship the pole (instead of God) with offerings and incense (2 Kings 18:4). They mistakenly believed that the power to heal came from the bronze pole and not from God. Of course, things never went well when the Israelites neglected God and worshipped idols. Eventually, King Hezekiah smashed the pole so that the Israelites could no longer burn incense to it.

The image of the snake-entwined pole carried over into Greek and Roman mythology. Those civilizations worshipped Asclepius, their pagan god of healing and medicine. Statues of Asclepius showed him carrying a snake-wrapped staff. Temples to honour this god were built all over the Mediterranean area and still existed when Jesus walked the earth. People paid to access medical services, which included bloodletting, walking around in the winter without shoes, and other practices, many of which did more harm than good. Asclepius was a counterfeit god.

There's a lesson in all that history. As Christians, we can value the healing power of today's beneficial medical care, but we shouldn't worship or idolize modern medicine as a god. We must recognize that the power to heal ultimately derives from God Himself, even when He chooses to guide us toward medical help.

Here's another matter worth addressing. While we must give due respect to medical professionals, we must be aware that such professionals don't always give reciprocal respect to Christian beliefs. Some medical professionals think of Christian healing practices as deluded, primitive, superstitious rites that have no place in our modern, educated society. We must not allow their views to discourage us. Thankfully, some doctors and medical researchers believe that faith has a constructive role to play in a person's health outcome.

Along with putting medical help into right balance and perspective, we can also put what medical specialists tell us into proper perspective. We can hear what they have to say (we should listen attentively), but we can remember that they are not the *final* authority on our diagnosis, treatment, or prognosis. God is. If a doctor gives us a negative prognosis, for example, we don't have to accept it unconditionally.

People diagnosed with cancer might be told that they likely have so many months or years to live. Doctors use their best judgment in making such statements, based on research statistics. Statistics have their proper place, but the medical outcomes of individuals don't always fall neatly into statistical probabilities. If a doctor says a person has a 10 percent chance of being alive within five years, what does that really mean? Who can say if the individual falls inside or outside of that 10 percent? The doctor has no way of knowing. Probabilities aren't certainties. The person shouldn't assume they fall into the doomed 90 percent.

Doctors sometimes use the word "incurable." I don't like that word. Jesus declared, "All things are possible" (Mark 9:23). Surely our all-knowing God can see possibility beyond what doctors can see. We can choose to see possibility too. We can believe that God can change our health situation, no matter how dismal it seems. The day will come when I will close my eyes and never open them again in this world, but until that day, I will trust in God's power to transform sickness back into health. I will hear, with due respect, what doctors tell me, but ultimately, I want to hear what God has to say about my health and potential healing. I'm not just a cold statistic to God. He alone knows what lies in store for me. He can still dispense hope when human doctors have run out of hope.

God has the power to put you or me in the coveted 10 percent (or 5 percent, or 1 percent) of those who will beat the morbid statistics. We must not let a statistic (or any other words spoken by a doctor) impose upon us a death sentence or a life sentence of unyielding sickness and suffering. God has the final say on how we will live and when we will die.

This brings to mind the story of David Kuo, who served as deputy director in the White House Office of Faith-Based and Community Initiatives. He fought cancer (both spiritually and through chemotherapy, radiation, and clinical trials). On three different occasions, doctors told him he had only six to twelve months left to live. David lived a decade after the first time he was given that prognosis. During those years, he fathered two children and wrote a book.[47]

Medication

Medication had a significant role to play in my recoveries from myositis, malaria, high blood pressure, and many other ailments over

the years. I'm thankful that we live in an age of advanced pharmaceutical aid.

When I talk with Christians who are against taking medication,
I present the simple scenario of a person afflicted with a headache.
Should that person pray for hours until God divinely heals their
headache? Why not also take fast-acting pain relief medication if it's
available? Is *that* wrong?

It's true that almost all drugs have side effects, risk of health
complications, and potential negative interactions with other drugs.
Medications have the power to both help and harm us. They are not
foolproof magic. We must proceed with wisdom and prudence. We
shouldn't rush to pop pills without duly assessing the risks versus
the benefits, but neither should we shun medications until we have
carefully assessed their worth. If we have concerns, we can discuss
them with our doctor and/or pharmacist.

God made many natural elements with inherent healing properties. The Bible provides clues to the medicinal properties of water,
soil, minerals, and plants. Humankind has learned how to use some of
those divinely created substances.

Consider these biblical examples of the healing power of water
and mud. Naaman was told to go bathe in the muddy Jordan River
to get rid of his leprosy (2 Kings 5:1–19). He obeyed and was healed.
Jesus healed a blind man by using mud, saliva, and water. Jesus "...
spit on the ground and made mud with the saliva. Then he anointed
the man's eyes with the mud and said to him, 'Go, wash in the pool of
Siloam'... So he went and washed and came back seeing" (John 9:6–7).
Jesus could have healed him by word or touch, but He chose to use a
mud potion and a water wash.

Mud has found its way into modern medicine. The well-known
antibacterial drug called penicillin was originally made from a fungus
(derived from soil) called penicillium. Some cutting-edge probiotics
contain soil-based organisms.

Medical scientists have discovered the healing properties of various earth minerals, which have been incorporated into medications,

supplements, and vitamins. Iron, for example, alleviates anemia. Zinc is added to ointments that treat wounds, creams that soothe eczema, and sunscreens that block the sun's ultraviolet rays.

The Bible reveals that some plants have healing properties. Isaiah applied a poultice of figs to King Hezekiah's boil (Isaiah 38:10–21). God used that natural therapy to heal the king. The trees of life in heaven have healing leaves (Revelation 22:2). Perhaps the Bible has inspired some scientists over the ages to investigate plant remedies. We now know that many plants have medicinal power. Morphine comes from poppy flowers. A heart drug, Digoxin, contains leaves from the *Digitalis purpurea* plant. Senna pods are crushed into many laxatives. Some blood pressure medications utilize reserpine roots. Cinchona bark is an ingredient in quinine, an element in many antimalarial drugs.

Pharmacologists, the pharmaceutical and vitamin industries, and naturopathic practitioners continue to gain knowledge about the healing effects of various minerals and plants and how they can be naturally used or beneficially synthetically altered.

Medical researchers are also learning more about how to harness the body's own healing mechanisms (designed by God). For example, they are now investigating the use of immunotherapy drugs, exploring how our immune systems can be boosted to successfully battle cancer cells. The immune system is supposed to search out cancer cells and destroy them before they can multiply. A healthy immune system comes equipped with "scout" cells (that roam the body looking for suspicious cells) and "soldier" cells (that can be called upon to fight invading cells). Sometimes cancer cells manipulate the immune system. Scout cells, tricked into accepting malignant cells as normal, don't alert soldier cells. The goal of immunotherapy is to reactivate the immobilized immune system so that it once again recognizes that cancer cells are abnormal and must be attacked. An optimally functioning immune system should be able to seek and destroy (or at least disable) invading cancer cells. In short, immunotherapy drugs help our natural immune system become more effective.

Immunotherapy is superior to chemotherapy in many ways: it's not toxic; it can search out straggler cells that surgery or radiation might have missed; and it can detect disease at the microscopic level before a visible tumour has developed. Immunotherapy is not usually used on its own yet. Doctors still have to rely on older methods, such as surgery (which cuts out cancer cells), chemotherapy (which poisons them), and radiation (which scorches them to death). Those three methods eliminate most cancer cells and then immunotherapy mops up what's left. Unfortunately, the three older methods adversely impact non-cancerous cells and can involve risks, complications, and nasty side effects.

Adding immunotherapy to the mix has already been demonstrated to improve survival rates for various cancers, including melanoma, bladder cancer, and colorectal cancer. As of 2016, over three hundred clinical trials were recruiting patients for immunotherapy in the U.S.

Former U.S. President Jimmy Carter developed melanoma that metastasized to the brain and liver. He was treated with immunotherapy in 2015. By year-end, Carter announced that doctors considered him cancer free.[48]

Let's be very grateful for such advances in medical research. God has allowed humankind to discover some of the wonderworking power inherent in His design of the body. Let's pray that God will further help medical scientists as they continue to develop newer, more targeted therapies to augment or replace old methods. Let's pray they discover therapies that are more efficient and less destructive to the body's healthy cells.

The present sad reality is that medication is not available for every ailment, nor is it effective in every situation. For decades, humankind has relied heavily on antibiotics to fight infections and various illnesses. Some superbugs (microbes such as bacteria, viruses, and parasites) now resist antibiotics. They've become stronger than the drugs that once treated them. In 2016, the United Nations General Assembly addressed the global problem of antimicrobial resistance. Treatment-resistant superbugs now kill about 700,000 people yearly.

The World Health Organization warns of a future post-antibiotic era, which would be "the end of modern medicine as we know it." If post-surgery infection cannot be treated, then surgery of any kind might become too risky.[49]

We cannot put our ultimate faith in antibiotics, or immunotherapy drugs, or any other medications. I'm thankful for the progress that research has made in treating various diseases, but there is still such a long way to go. I'm even *more* thankful that God has *perfect* understanding of each disease. Did you know that there are over two hundred kinds of cancer? I'm glad that God knows what has to happen in the body to fight each kind of cancer cell. Whether we're dealing with cancer or any other condition, we can pray that our doctor will have (or acquire) knowledge of existing drugs that can help us. If there's not yet a suitable medication, we can pray that, with God's help, one will be developed (or further developed). In the meantime, we can continue to pray for God's divine healing power to work in our bodies.

Tissues, Transplants, and Transfusions

The John 9:6–7 story, described earlier, illustrates the healing property of saliva, a body fluid. On another occasion:

> *...some people brought to him [Jesus] a man who was deaf and could hardly talk, and they begged Jesus to place his hand on him. After he took him aside, away from the crowd, Jesus put his fingers into the man's ears. Then he spit and touched the man's tongue. He looked up to heaven and with a deep sigh said to him, "Ephphatha!" (which means "Be opened!"). At this, the man's ears were opened, his tongue was loosened and he began to speak plainly.*
>
> Mark 7:32–35, NIV

In Mark 8:22–25, we read yet another story about Jesus using saliva. He placed it on a blind man's eyes, thereby healing him.

Do you think that those biblical stories encourage the use of one person's biological material to heal another? Medical science has learned how to utilize human tissue in organ transplants, blood transfusions, and certain vaccines. Donor tissue from one person can improve or even save another life.

I've known a few people whose organs (liver or lungs) were seriously failing. They became the recipients of donated organs that saved their lives and eventually restored their health.

Physical Therapy

The Bible alludes to the power that is released when one human being simply touches another. Jesus frequently used His touch to heal people (see, for example, Mark 7:31–3; 8:22–25). We've already talked about the prayerful laying on of hands, which allows God's supernatural power to flow through human hands.

What about the modern practices of massage, chiropractic therapy, physiotherapy, and other healing methods, which recognize the therapeutic benefit of human touch? I believe God can use those adjunct natural therapies to effect some measure of healing (although they are *not* the same thing as the Spirit-empowered practice of laying hands on a sick person).

Surgery

At times, we may need surgery. I had to have surgery when my inflamed appendix burst at the age of fourteen, spreading poisonous infection through my abdomen. I most recently had gallbladder surgery. Perhaps you've experienced surgery too.

Jesus put His fingers *into* a man's ears in the process of healing him (Mark 7:31–35). This was an intrusive form of healing. Was that a foreshadow of doctors putting their hands into the patient's incised body during the course of surgery?

I've seen God bless surgery in the lives of many friends. One woman, for example, could barely walk because of excruciating pain in both hips. Hip replacements have restored her mobility. I'm happy to see how often she walks, travels, and golfs.

Sometimes we have the luxury of time to pray about whether or not to undergo surgery. If the surgery is elective, we can wait until we have peace.

At times, I have chosen not to have surgery. Just before my first child was born, I endured labour for about thirty-two hours. At the twenty-four-hour point, my obstetrician and an anaesthetist spoke with me. They said they were preparing the operating room for a C-section procedure. This came as a total surprise. I asked if either the baby or I were in imminent danger. We were not. The doctors simply thought I'd been in labour long enough. The anaesthetist, who was finishing his shift soon, announced that the medical team was already "sharpening the knives." I told him that I would only consent to a C-section if it became necessary for the health and safety of either my baby or myself. Then I continued labour for another eight hours before a successful natural birth.

I don't mean to discourage others from having *necessary* C-sections. Nor do I want to make anyone feel bad because they've already had one. My point is that surgery is often elective and not absolutely necessary. We must seek God's wisdom and guidance. Like medication, surgery carries risks of complications and adverse outcomes. The perceived benefits must outweigh the risks. We must be at peace before we proceed.

God Being God

Every once in a while, God has shown me that He can heal a person before a medical professional has the opportunity to do anything. For twenty-five years, my husband, Sam, worked as a youth camp doctor for a week or two every summer. One July day, a skateboarder at the camp took a bad fall and injured his shoulder. My husband could see and feel that the shoulder was badly dislocated. A group of five medical staff gathered around the boy and began praying. Before Sam could attempt to put the joint back in place, it suddenly went back into its socket all on its own, without manipulation. The boy got up and declared he was no longer in pain. Getting back on his skateboard, he sped away.

A relative of mine had his own experience of God being God in the midst of a medical situation. One winter about eight years ago, this healthy man in his fifties suddenly and inexplicably lost power in his left hand. He had trouble buttoning his shirt, tying shoelaces, combing his hair, and performing other ordinary tasks. Alternating tingling and numbness soon developed, followed by pain radiating from his neck down to his left arm.

Over the next few months, he received *eight* different medical opinions from seven different doctors, all of them highly respected in their fields. The first doctor told him he was likely suffering from a pinched nerve, which might require surgery. The second doctor, a specialist at a leading hospital, diagnosed myasthenia gravis (a serious neuromuscular disease). The third doctor, a prominent surgeon, recommended spinal surgery to deal with nerve root issues, while additionally opining that this relative might have Amyotrophic Lateral Sclerosis, also known as ALS (a neurological disease that usually results in a cruel death process within a few years of onset). A neurologist later told my relative that he had Multiple Sclerosis (MS), a different neurological disease. Other doctors diagnosed post-viral vasculitis and post-viral encephalopathy. It was a perplexing, frustrating, and frightening time for my relative.

The various specialists performed a variety of diagnostic tests, including blood work, X-rays, CT scans, and MRIs. While the doctors were still trying to figure out the situation, my relative was healed. His symptoms disappeared and never came back. He was relieved that he didn't require surgery or have to cope with a serious disease like ALS. His spontaneous healing had no explanation apart from God directing the healing process.

God works through doctors, other professionals, and various medical means, but He also likes to clearly show us, from time to time, that He is the supreme Healer.

In conclusion, we should respect doctors and value their extensive training and experience. We must be immensely grateful whenever we have the opportunity to consult them, but we shouldn't worship the ground they walk on. We need to keep in mind the limitations of their humanity. We can take medication and undergo surgery or other therapy, when warranted, but let's always remember that God is our true Healer. Just as God graciously healed people while Moses lifted up a metal pole, and Jesus healed some people by using means such as mud, water, or saliva, God can still use human and earthly resources in the healing process today. (After all, He created those physical resources and the brilliant minds of medical researchers and practitioners.) No matter *how* we are healed, God must get the final credit for restored health and sustained life.

22

_____

SEEK (AND OFFER) PRACTICAL SUPPORT

I will always value those family members and friends who have ministered to me in my seasons of illness. I remember their kindness, support, and tender-loving care. They sat with me. They brought food, drink, and medicine to my bedside. I can still hear echoes of the prayers they prayed for me.

The story that Jesus told about the Good Samaritan demonstrates that we are to care for those in physical need. That well-known story (found in Luke 10:30–37) opens with a man walking from Jerusalem to Jericho. Bandits attacked him, beating him severely. They left him unclothed by the roadside, half-dead. A priest and a Levite came down that road. They cruelly crossed to the other side after seeing the stricken man. A Samaritan man then came along. With compassion, the Samaritan tended to the wounds of the injured man. Then the Samaritan let the victim ride on his own animal to an inn, where he took further care of him. The next day, the Samaritan paid the innkeeper, in advance, to take ongoing care of the recovering man, promising to pay more on his return trip. Jesus instructed His followers to act mercifully like the Good Samaritan (v. 37).

On another occasion, Jesus declared that when we minister to the sick, we are, in effect, ministering to Him (Matthew 25:34–40).

He promised that those who care for others in need will inherit His kingdom.

I think of my parents coming to visit me during the five weeks I spent in the hospital as a nine-year-old child. They came a long distance, even though they knew they couldn't stay more than a few minutes because they had to leave my older sister downstairs watching my younger twin brothers. (Child siblings weren't allowed in patient wards in those days.) My parents brought me my favourite foods because I was no fan of the barely palatable hospitable food that was served back then.

Years later, my sister helped me when I was sick with malaria in India. She worked hard to keep me hydrated, especially during hours of high fevers. Our hotel room tap water wasn't safe to drink, and in those days, it wasn't easy to find clean bottled water. She rode around town in a tuk-tuk to find a chemist's shop, to get advice about my condition, and to buy medication to treat me.

I remember my husband nursing me in a hotel room in a small Turkish town after a severe case of food poisoning struck me. He stayed up with me during that first horrible night. He brought me tea and encouraged me to drink it a sip at a time. The next day, he brought soup when I could bear it. I felt like a child again.

When I developed severe pain from a blocked gallbladder, Sam brought me to our local hospital before dawn's light. He stayed up during the night to pray while I underwent emergency surgery, and he was at my side when I was wheeled from the recovery room into my hospital room. He later drove me home, picked up my medications from the pharmacy, taxied me around while I was on narcotic pain relief, and took over some of my duties. He made sure I received timely and appropriate follow-up care when he realized my recovery wasn't progressing smoothly.

When our health suffers, we must humble ourselves to ask for and receive human help on a very practical level. And, of course, we must be thankful for it.

We might also need support while being the caregiver of a loved one. A neighbour offered to watch my young daughter many days after school so I could be with my son when he was in the hospital. A dear friend brought dinner to my front door when another family member was in the hospital. Friends have come to hospital rooms to visit the patient, but also to keep company with those of us who spent hours by the patient's bedside. Those friends treated me to cups of coffee and meals at just the right times. They stayed with my ailing loved one while I got out for a walk. I thank God for those who know how to minister to the sick *and* their caregivers.

My church community knows how to minister well. An army of helpers can be mobilized to: drive sick persons to medical appointments; sit with them through procedures such as chemotherapy; cook and deliver meals to them and their families; run errands for them; keep up gardening and home maintenance; and take over communicating the status of a patient for an exhausted family. I have seen this in action, particularly for those dealing with a serious cancer diagnosis over a long period. This level of ministry is something to behold.

Like those willing servants, we can look for ways to offer practical support to the sick, the suffering, and the recovering. Beyond the suggestions just mentioned, we can give money to help with medical expenses that government programs or insurance policies might not cover, such as the small fortune it costs to park at an urban hospital.

One relative lay in a hospital bed hour upon hour, day after day, unable to sit up or walk. With drainage tubes coming out of his chest, and with his body hooked up to oxygen and intravenous lines, he couldn't even roll over. His skin began to deteriorate, most noticeably on his feet. When I talked with a nurse about that, she left the room and came back with a basin of warm water and a washcloth. I found myself washing this patient's feet. It was an act of humility and servanthood, wordlessly communicating that I cared. Jesus washed the feet of His disciples. As I followed His example that day, I hoped that my relative could feel the compassion of Christ flowing through me.

I know that I profoundly experienced the presence of Christ in that simple act of service.

Tender-loving care is highly therapeutic. It can play a significant role in recovery from illness, injury, or surgery. I encourage you to ask for practical help when you're in need, but to be equally ready to offer it when you're well. God's healing power flowed through the Good Samaritan's practical help. It can flow through us too.

23

CHOOSE PATIENCE AND PERSEVERANCE

One Easter Sunday some years ago, a loved one wasn't well. At church that morning, I heard the glorious Easter message. I felt uplifted for a while, but after church, I began moping around. If God could raise Christ from the dead, why hadn't He healed my loved one? Jesus lay in the tomb for three days. My loved one had been suffering intermittently for three years. It was growing harder to sustain faith, trust, and hope.

I was busy in my home that afternoon when I felt an inner nudging to turn on the television. Those who know me well can appreciate how strange an impulse that was. My family can attest that I rarely turn on the television and almost never watch programs alone. My husband rules the remote control. I watch a handful of shows each week that my husband and I both enjoy. He does all the necessary clicking.

None of our favourite shows aired on Sunday afternoons, so I ignored the unusual impulse. The inner prompting grew more insistent. Finally, I gave in and began to surf channels (which I *never* do). One program arrested my attention. A man was testifying about how God had healed him of the same health problem that plagued my loved one.

I listened to the man intently. He had suffered for a *dozen* years. He had prayed and prayed, to no seeming avail. One day, with the last bit of faith he had left, he went forward to the front of his church for healing prayer. After that day, his illness never recurred.

After hearing that story, my first thought was this: I did not want to wait a dozen years for God to answer my family's prayers. Our loved one had already gone forward for prayer at the front of more than one church. I asked God: Are we really going to have to keep waiting? Deep within, I sensed God assuring me that He doesn't work in quite the same timing, or the same way, from one person to the next. We wouldn't necessarily have to wait another nine years for our loved one to be healed. But I *did* get the clear impression that we would have to wait for *some* period of time. We were going to have to be patient. We were going to have to persevere in our faith.

From time to time, I remembered the man's testimony on that Easter Sunday program. Sometimes I fussed and fumed about the waiting process, but then I would resolve afresh to carry on with patient perseverance. God would answer our ongoing prayers for healing in a manner and at a time of *His* choosing. I didn't have any choice in the matter.

I felt that God had given me a sign that Easter Sunday, just as He had given King Hezekiah a sign (2 Kings 20:8–11). That passage reveals that God heard the king's prayer for healing and, in response, promised to heal him. For whatever reason, God didn't heal him immediately. Instead, He gave King Hezekiah a sign: God would cause the shadow on the ground outside to retreat backwards ten steps. It has never made much sense to me that God would use His power to make the sun travel backwards instead of using that power to make King Hezekiah instantly well. Why give a sign to the king instead of healing him straightaway? God doesn't always make sense from our human point of view. God healed the king at the time He chose. After some years, He substantially healed my loved one too.

I've heard people say: "God didn't heal me (or my loved one) of (whatever)." It sounds like they've given up. Others say: "God hasn't healed me *yet*." That statement suggests that the speaker hasn't lost faith, trust, and hope. Instead, they're pressing on. They're still *waiting* for God to heal them. What have you been saying about your health predicament? Who enjoys waiting? Not me. Few of us are naturally patient. Our modern trend of seeking instant gratification doesn't help.

Over twenty times in the Psalms, the question "how long?" gets asked. That's a question that might rumble around in our heads when confronted with sustained sickness or suffering. How long is this going to last? When is it going to end?

Addressing the two human tendencies to be impatient and give up too easily, the apostle Paul wrote: "We do not want you to become lazy, but to imitate those who through faith and patience inherit what has been promised" (Hebrews 6:12, NIV).

In Romans 8:24b–25, Paul tied hope and patience together: "Now hope that is seen is not hope. For who hopes for what he sees? But if we hope for what we do not see, we wait for it with patience."

One psalmist linked faith with patience when he scribed: "Yet I am confident I will see the Lord's goodness while I am here in the land of the living. Wait patiently for the Lord. Be brave and courageous…" (Psalm 27:13–14, NLT).

When reading gospel accounts of Jesus healing people, we might assume that the healings were instant. Many of the people He healed had been sick or disabled for a long time, such as the invalid by the Pool of Bethsaida, who had been waiting to be healed for thirty-eight years (John 5:2–9). Jesus healed the invalid the very day He met him at the pool. In one sense, the healing was instant, but we don't know the backstory to that healing. How many prayers had that man prayed over thirty-eight years? How many priests had he implored to pray? Had the invalid appealed to God, over and over, on the basis of Old Testament scriptures about healing? Had the invalid heard about Jesus long before the day of his healing? Was he aware of the growing reputation that Jesus had for healing the sick? Had he heard about specific healings? Had faith arisen in him, way back then, that God might heal him one day? Had he asked God to send Jesus his way? Had Jesus ever been to the Pool of Bethsaida before, healing others? Had those healings stirred his own faith that it could happen to him too? From the invalid's point of view, his healing might have felt a long time coming.

Think about the many other people Jesus healed at a certain point in time. Had they also prayed in advance? Had they heard about Jesus and His miracles beforehand? Had they followed Jesus, day after day? Had they tried to press through the crowds on earlier occasions to get close to Jesus?

At a minimum, many individuals probably followed Jesus all day long to get near Him. We know that great crowds often surrounded Jesus. For example, when Jesus got off a boat one day, after crossing the Sea of Galilee, a "large crowd followed and pressed around him" (Mark 5:24, NIV). Pressing suggests some jostling, pushing, and shoving, everyone trying to get as close as they could.

Getting near Jesus was no doubt harder than getting the autograph of a rockstar. Perhaps you've seen old footage of when the Beatles first came to America in the 1960s. Hysterical mobs of adoring fans pressed in to get closer. Once the fame of Jesus had spread far and wide, I imagine that a similar mob scene occurred whenever He arrived in a town. A person would really have to persevere in their efforts to get right beside Jesus. Maybe they were able to do that the first day they tried. Maybe not. Maybe they had to wait a while before Jesus returned again to minister in their town.

Not long before I wrote this chapter, I had the opportunity to meet Mark Burnett, executive producer of popular reality shows on television, such as "Survivor," "Apprentice," and "Shark Tank." I had to wait in a crowd for my turn to speak with him. I would never have had the opportunity to meet him had I just circled the perimeter of the crowd. No, I had to press in (politely of course). I had to patiently wait. I had to persevere.

We know that many people followed Jesus from one town to another. Matthew 12:15–16, for example, reports: "… Jesus withdrew from that place. A large crowd followed him, and he healed all who were ill…" (NIV). Those people chose patience and persistence. They didn't give up.

In one village, after sunset, the "whole town gathered at the door" of the home where Jesus was staying (Mark 1:32–34). The crowd included everyone who was sick. Jesus healed many of them, but not all. Those who weren't healed probably had to try again some other time, when they could get closer to Him. Maybe they followed Him on foot to the next few villages.

After describing one large crowd that "followed Jesus and pressed around him," the Gospel of Mark mentions a woman who somehow managed to get through the crowd, close enough to Jesus to reach out and touch Him:

> And there was a woman who had had a discharge of blood for
> twelve years... She had heard the reports about Jesus and came up
> behind him in the crowd and touched his garment. For she said, "If
> I touch even his garments, I will be made well." And immediately
> the flow of blood dried up, and she felt in her body that she was
> healed of her disease. And Jesus, perceiving in himself that power
> had gone out from him, immediately turned about in the crowd
> and said, "Who touched my garments?" And his disciples said to
> him, "You see the crowd pressing around you, and yet you say,
> 'Who touched me?'"
>
> Mark 5:25, 27–31

The woman who touched Jesus was determined to find healing. She must have been anemic and weak after losing so much blood for so long. That makes her tenacity in pressing through the crowd to get to Jesus all the more remarkable. Faith must have been building up in her since she first heard reports of other healings.

I suspect there's a backstory for most of the healings we read about in scripture. I doubt that most people *first* thought of asking Jesus (or one of His followers) for healing two seconds before they came forward. Yes, most were healed on the specific day that Jesus prayed over them or laid His hands on them, but there might have been a long history of persistent prayer and growing faith preceding that moment of healing.

Thankfully, in our era, we don't have to physically press in to meet Jesus, or follow Him from place to place, or wait until we have a spot at the front of the line to tell Him about our needs. He's always just a prayer away. His Spirit dwells within believers all the time. But we *do* have to be patient and persevering in waiting for His response to our prayers. We have to *spiritually* press on and press in.

Many times we may feel that healing is happening two steps forward, one step back (or one step forward, three steps back). In such times, we must still press on and press in, putting one foot in front of the next, moving forward as best we can.

Jesus told His disciples that "they should always pray and not give up" (Luke 18:1, NIV). On that same occasion, Jesus told them a parable about a widow who persisted in coming to a judge, asking for justice. The judge refused until finally the widow's persistence wore him down. Unlike that human judge, God does not need to be worn down, but God values and rewards persistence.

Healing is often a process, sometimes a long one. God might heal a person one bout of illness at a time, with periods of good health in between. But they should never give up asking for a greater measure of healing. God finally healed the man who testified on the Easter Sunday television program. He had doggedly persisted in praying for complete healing, not just healing of each recurring flare-up of his disease.

Waiting with patience and perseverance is not a passive exercise. We must be active in the spiritual realm while we're waiting, doing the various things discussed in this book. Even if we lay, day after day, in a sickbed, we can still pray, meditate on His words, choose faith and trust, praise Him, and seek intercession from others. Seeking healing is not for the faint of heart or weak of will. We must not allow ourselves to grow weary. We need grit. We need determination. We must resolve to go the distance.

Let me tell you more about the Dutch man named Brother Andrew. He began missionary training college in 1953. Soon after, he developed some slipped discs in his back. Sometimes the consequent pain was so bad, he could barely comb his hair or dress himself. At times, he had trouble walking or even standing. When the pain was *really* bad, he spent weeks in bed.

Doctors couldn't help him. They told him that back surgery was too risky. Other Christians prayed for him, anointed him with oil, and laid their hands on him. Although Brother Andrew trusted in God for healing, the debilitating back flare-ups continued. At times, they were excruciating.

Despite the pain, he began to travel far and wide, focusing on the needs of others. He had fully surrendered his life to God, and he meant to keep his commitment to go anywhere and do anything God wanted.

He began his well-known ministry, serving underground persecuted churches, in 1955. God led him to smuggle Bibles into countries such as Czechoslovakia, Russia, and Poland, which were, at that time, behind the formidable Iron Curtain. At great risk to his own life, Brother Andrew travelled to those Communist countries, delivering Bibles and other forbidden Christian literature. He encouraged his Christian brothers and sisters wherever he found them.

Forming an organization called Open Doors, Brother Andrew gathered other Christians to help him strengthen the churches in the Soviet bloc. He wrote an inspiring book about his work in Eastern Europe titled *God's Smuggler*.[50]

While reaching out to persecuted brothers and sisters in other nations, Brother Andrew continued to suffer with severe back pain for *eighteen* years. He remained patient as he waited for his healing. He kept busy with his ministry work during all those years.

In 1971, God finally healed Brother Andrew in a most unorthodox way. Brother Andrew had agreed to fly to Denver with a pilot friend. Shortly after take-off, the small plane crashed, breaking two vertebrae in Brother Andrew's lower back. You can imagine the additional pain that put him in. His back was in worse shape than ever. He remained in hospital for two weeks, then spent further months in recovery. For a few months, he had to wear a rigid plaster cast that started just below his arms and went down to his hips.

His wife came over from Holland to be with him. She read Bible passages to him every day, sometimes for hours. Famed faith healer Kathryn Kuhlman prayed for him, and so did the hospital chaplain. Countless supporters around the world prayed for him.

Months after the plane crash, Brother Andrew finally shed his cast and gradually renewed his strength. In the end, *all* of his back pain disappeared. God completely healed him. After eighteen years of back pain, he never had trouble with slipped discs again. He began to play tennis and golf, run, garden, and bicycle—activities he could only dream of before his plane crash.[51]

Over the decades since that healing, Brother Andrew has expanded his organization's ministry to other continents. Open Doors smuggled one million Bibles into China on a single night, offloading the precious cargo from a barge anchored in darkness off the coast. After the Soviet empire's collapse, Brother Andrew received permission to legally deliver one million Bibles into Russia. Not so legally, he and his organization have taken Bibles into countries such as Afghanistan, Iran, and even Saudi Arabia. Their present mission focuses on persecuted Muslim-background believers. Brother Andrew has learned to apply the same patience and perseverance in his ministry that he developed while waiting for healing.

My daughter-in-law experienced a season of waiting during one of her pregnancies. In her second trimester, she was diagnosed with placenta previa. After bleeding at week twenty-four, she wisely went to the hospital. The doctors told her to take it easy. She started bleeding again at week twenty-six. After going to the local emergency unit, she was transferred by ambulance to a hospital specializing in premature birth care. The medical specialists there told her that they might have to do an emergency C-section if the bleeding got worse. This could become necessary to save her life. She could die if she hemorrhaged too much. The doctors also gave her a steroid shot in case they had to deliver the baby prematurely. She learned that an infant born that early would have many medical problems *if* they survived.

My daughter-in-law remained in hospital for a week. She was discharged with instructions to maintain strict bed or couch rest for the final trimester of her pregnancy. The doctors hoped that her pregnancy would last for further weeks.

She prayed as one nail-biting day slowly followed another. Her church prayed. Her family prayed, along with friends and other intercessors.

God gave her the verse: "Be still, and know that I am God" (Psalm 46:10a). She had no real choice. Under doctors' orders, she had to be still. She had to be patient. She had to *wait*. The timing of her baby's birth remained in God's hands.

I admire my daughter-in-law for the faith-filled patience she daily demonstrated during her final trimester, sitting on a couch or laying on her bed. Her pregnancy lasted until week thirty-eight (which is considered full term), and our awesome little grandson was born, healthy and strong. She would surely agree that her time of patiently being still was well worth it!

24

Manage Thoughts and Feelings

Sports psychologists train athletes to be mentally and emotionally tough so that they don't break under pressure. Athletes learn how to sometimes push through pain. God, through His Word and other means, can train us to be mentally and emotionally tough so that we don't break under pressure or pain while awaiting healing.

I suspect that some readers might be struggling, mentally and emotionally, while trying to cope with a health issue. Perhaps you're one of them. Perhaps your sickness, disability, injury, or long recovery has led to a mudslide of anger, fear, worry, frustration, confusion, self-pity, discouragement, depression, or other hard-to-deal-with thoughts and feelings. Maybe they overwhelm you sometimes. It's normal to experience those states of heart and mind. I don't judge you. I understand. I have travelled through undesirable inner territory when confronted with health issues. I feel compassion for you. I know that God does too. I wish I could give you a hug. I cannot do that for most of you, but I can point you toward the help that God has to offer.

Our daily choice of thoughts and emotions can affect us physically. Medical research has discovered the significant interconnection between our mental health, emotional health, and physical health. Good thoughts and feelings, such as joy and peace, have a positive impact on us physically. Finding joy in the Lord strengthens us (Nehemiah 8:10). Other kinds of thoughts and feelings are destructive to our physical wellbeing. Anger, anxiety, and depression are particularly notorious for adverse impact on physical health. Chronic anger has been linked to fatigue, muscle aches, digestive disorders, headaches, insomnia, cardiac problems, and even cancer. Sustained anxiety contributes to gastrointestinal issues, asthma, skin problems, a weakened immune system, and many other health concerns.[52]

A negative mental/emotional pattern *might* be *one* of the reasons we're sick in the first place. Or it might explain why we're not progressing to full recovery. Of course, our thoughts and feelings aren't usually the *only* reason that medical problems develop or persist. I want to make that very clear. We can also develop illness as a result of such factors as our genetic make-up, exposure to chemical toxins, contact with harmful bacteria and viruses, and lifestyle choices related to diet, exercise, sleep, alcohol, drugs, and cigarettes.

Even if negative thoughts and feelings aren't the primary reason for our sickness or slow recovery, they can exacerbate our physical health problems. A person might develop high blood pressure, for example, because of hereditary factors, a sedentary lifestyle, too much salt in their diet, and advancing age. Chronic issues such as anger or anxiety might not have caused that person's high blood pressure, but such mental and emotional states are not friendly to that medical condition.

Bringing Our Thoughts Captive

Our emotions are usually triggered by our thoughts. If you don't like what you're feeling and expressing, pause to examine what you're thinking. We can get a grip on our feelings by bringing our thoughts under the control of our will. Paul instructed believers to "take captive every thought to make it obedient to Christ" (2 Corinthians 10:5, NIV). On another occasion, Paul urged believers to be "transformed" by the "renewal" of their minds (Romans 12:2).

We can decide to stop thinking the kind of thoughts that generate anger, worry, despair, self-pity, or other undesirable inner states. Instead, we can choose to focus our minds on thoughts that generate love, forgiveness, faith, trust, hope, peace, joy, and gratitude. We can make choices, moment by moment. We cannot be in both positive and negative mental territory at the same time.

Hundreds of Bible verses can help to direct our thoughts. Meditating on God's words can renew our minds. Positive thoughts and feelings can help our recovery. Proverbs 14:30 states: "A tranquil heart gives life to the flesh…" Proverbs 17:22 declares: "A cheerful heart is good medicine…" (NIV).

We might spend our entire lives trying to better manage our inner selves. It's not a quick and easy process. *This* moment is a good time to get a fresh grip on our thoughts and feelings. Tomorrow will require further effort.

If you're interested in the topic of managing thoughts and emotions according to biblical principles, I invite you to read my book *Bent Out of Shape*.[53] It contains more than five hundred verses pertaining to thoughts and feelings. It discusses how we can practically move from negative, health-impairing states such as anger, anxiety, and depression, to health-enhancing states such as love, forgiveness, and contentment.

Praying for Emotional Healing

Some people have been emotionally traumatized, perhaps by a health crisis or by situations such as sexual abuse, a messy divorce, a serious accident, or a toxic workplace. Severe trauma can impact physical health.

We might need prayer for emotional healing as much as we need prayer for physical healing. Some people discover that once their emotional issues have been dealt with, their physical symptoms begin to dissipate. We can ask God to heal both body *and* soul. God "heals the brokenhearted and binds up their wounds" (Psalm 147:3). The wounds might produce scars, but they will fade over time. Counselling sessions with a pastor, medical doctor, psychologist, or psychiatrist can augment prayer for the healing of our souls.

Sooner or later, if others caused our trauma, we must address the issue of forgiving them. Forgiveness can help us to get rid of anger, resentment, and bitterness. If we caused our own trauma (perhaps as the driver who caused a car accident), we can get rid of guilt, shame, and self-condemnation by receiving God's forgiveness, followed by forgiving ourselves.

I recall attending a session at a healing conference that dealt specifically with the power of forgiveness. Prayer was offered for those wanting to forgive others or themselves. Many people later reported healing of longstanding medical issues, especially chronic pain, after they had dealt with unforgiveness.

Some people have a root of rejection anchored deep in their soul. They might have felt rejected by parents (especially if they were abandoned), by a spouse (especially if they are divorced), by teachers, friends, dates, or work colleagues. If others have rejected them, they might also reject themselves. This can impact their health on every level (physical, mental, emotional, and spiritual).

Some people reject their own bodies because of their size, skin colour, or any other aspect of their appearance. We must learn to love our own bodies. God designed and created them and has chosen to dwell within them.

Whatever caused a root of self-rejection to grow within, we can ask God to emotionally heal us.

When a Loved One Is Sick or Suffering

We might struggle with tough emotions when a loved one has a health problem. We might have to work through sadness, worry, or discouragement. If a family member is sick for a long time, their caregiver might begin to resent them, especially if the caregiver has sacrificed elements of their own life. A caregiver might also be resentful if they think that the illness or injury arose from the ailing person's own fault (for example, from risky behaviour, smoking, drinking in excess, or not taking medication). I have not yet experienced that kind of resentment, but I suspect that we all have the capacity to be resentful if caregiving goes on for a long time. We could also develop self-pity or depression.

If we want to help our ailing loved ones on the mental and emotional level, we must do the hard work of dealing with our *own* unhelpful thoughts and feelings. When we serve by a sickbed, let us resolve to be like those described in Psalm 84:6a: "When they walk through the Valley of Weeping, it will become a place of refreshing springs" (NLT). Imagine being a refreshing spring to a loved one in physical distress.

Let's decide to be His heart, voice, hands, and feet. Let's ask Him to guide and empower our prayers, words, and actions. Let's be bearers of God's love, kindness, compassion, empathy, mercy, and grace as we come alongside those who need healing.

Love is most important. Jesus advised that the second greatest commandment (after the command to love God) is to love others as we love ourselves (Matthew 22:39). Most doctors will agree that loving care assists the healing process.

Feeling Overwhelmed

During times of sickness, injury, or surgery, our world can feel out of control. We must not let a health challenge ruin our whole lives. We must resist feeling overwhelmed by the inner and outer disorder that can so quickly engulf us in times of health crisis. God can help us control the chaos.

Ships are designed to have several compartments. One part of a ship can be disabled without affecting the other compartments. If one section gets flooded with water, or is on fire, tightly sealed doors can be quickly shut, isolating that area. The watertight and flameproof doors prevent flood or fire from spreading beyond the sealed compartment. In other areas of the ship, life can go on as normally as possible.

I was once on a cruise ship at sea when a fire started on board. Over the loudspeaker, the captain announced the fire, assuring everyone it was under control. Metal barriers had indeed closed off a section of the ship, containing the fire. Only emergency responders could stay in there. Thousands of passengers carried on with planned activities in other areas. I was impressed by how effectively the captain prevented chaos.

When a medical crisis happens, we can secure the health compartment of our lives, as much as we are able to, so that the crisis doesn't automatically spill over into other areas of our lives. We shouldn't let illness or injury *unduly* impact our marriages, other relationships, careers, finances, or unrelated aspects of our health. Of course, there might be *some* impact we cannot avoid, but let's resist *whatever* amount of collateral damage we can. This will help us to manage our innermost selves.

It's important not to let our whole lives descend into chaos. Children still need to be cared for, homes cleaned, bills paid, laundry done, meals cooked. If we cannot take care of these matters, we can ask for help or pay for it. Some things may have to go on the back burner for a while, but not everything has to fall apart. My writing, for example, has been interrupted by illnesses and hospitalizations, but necessary matters have been taken care of.

This is often easier said than done. When illness, injury, or surgery beset our world, our minds are often swirling in circles like hurricane winds. Even if we're not the sick or recovering one, our lives can easily be turned upside down when a loved one isn't well. Caregivers must also make sure they resist chaos and collateral damage in their lives. Caregivers need rest and refreshment if they're going to go the distance. That's not being selfish. That's being wise.

When Sam was in the hospital with a brain bleed, I had to put all of this into practice. I forced myself to leave the hospital in the early evening to go home for a proper meal. I answered emails and called supportive people. I took time to read my Bible and pray in the quieter atmosphere of my own home. I tried to maintain some exercise routines. I made time for my adult children. This helped me manage my thoughts and feelings. I wasn't being callous or uncaring. I knew that the medical situation wouldn't resolve quickly. There was no point letting my whole life fall apart. I was going to have to be strong and supportive for *months*, not days, as Sam's brain slowly recovered.

While dealing with matters that had to be addressed at Sam's office while he was still off work, I kept reminding myself of the words of Paul: "I can do all this through him [Jesus] who gives me strength" (Philippians 4:13, NIV). During that stressful time, I learned that I could indeed do everything I needed to do, with the strength of Christ working in me. God helped me to stay calm and focused. With His help, I was daily astonished at how I was able to keep putting one foot in front of the other, getting everything done. I didn't feel alone, even when I was alone.

I encouraged my kids to resist any collateral damage. They rushed to the ICU as soon as they heard about their dad's brain bleed. Our daughter had been writing December law school exams at an out-of-town university. She missed an exam the day she came. A few days later, she asked me if she should stay and miss further exams. I knew that would create chaos in her life. She'd already been told she would have to make up any missed exams. I encouraged her to get her exams over with. That first week of his hospitalization, Sam was asleep much of the time, or he was away from his hospital room getting tests done. After going back to university, she kept in close touch with her dad and me over the phone. She soon came home for a few weeks over Christmas and spent quality time with her dad, who later agreed that she'd made the right decision.

Jesus commanded: "… Love your neighbor as yourself" (Matthew 22:39, NIV). We must love our family members and friends when they are ailing, but we must take the time to appropriately love (and take care of) our own selves.

The Power of Encouragement

How can we find encouragement during a health crisis? One way is to remember God's past faithfulness. Recalling the great works God had performed in their collective past encouraged the Israelites. One psalmist wrote: "I will meditate on your majestic, glorious splendor and your wonderful miracles" (Psalm 145:5, NLT). We can remember our own healing stories and those of friends and family members.

God might encourage us by bringing someone across our path to uplift us. I heard a speaker at the National Conference of Leading Women in 2008. She was the Dean of Students at a prominent Christian university. Her husband, a doctor who treated patients during the SARS crisis in Toronto, contracted SARS himself and almost died. (SARS is the acronym for a viral illness called Severe Acute Respiratory Syndrome.) Her husband spent eight months as a patient in the hospital and lost eighty-seven pounds. He was in a coma for a while. God eventually healed him. The conference speaker talked about how her devotional life (prayer and Bible study) infused her with daily courage during her husband's long ordeal. By sharing her story, she encouraged me.

We can read faith-inspiring books about healing. I've already mentioned some books written by Francis MacNutt. He has studied the subject of healing for many decades and has prayed for countless people who have been healed. For years, he has run Christian Healing Ministries (based in Florida) and has travelled far and wide to speak on the topic of healing.

MacNutt started out believing that healing always had to be a miraculous, extraordinary occurrence. He thought that only saints could pray for healing. He didn't claim to be a saint, so he didn't feel qualified to pray for healing or to expect that God would hear his prayers. Over time, his academic research (on church history) convinced him that healing should be a normal, ordinary experience in the Christian life and that *all* Christians could step out to access God's healing power for themselves or others.[54]

As he stepped out in faith to pray for the sick, he saw how often God answered his prayers. In the first thirty years of his healing ministry, MacNutt claims to have seen thousands of people healed.[55] (He says that, of course, we can't absolutely prove that a healing took place because of prayer, or solely because of prayer, but he asserts that the number of people who have been healed after being prayed for is certainly noteworthy.) MacNutt's personal journey and his stories about others have encouraged me.

Sometimes we can just sit back and marvel when God directly intervenes in a situation with His encouraging presence. During my husband's hospital stay for the treatment of a brain bleed, he spent his first week in the ICU. Night seven was rough. When his nurse stepped away from her post at the edge of his cubicle, Sam got up on his own to walk to the bathroom. He fell and hurt himself. The rest of the night went downhill from there. Discouraged, Sam wondered if he wanted to continue living.

When I arrived at the hospital the next morning, Sam was sitting quietly, hunched over in a chair. There was no light in his blank eyes. His spirit seemed strangely absent from his body. He mouthed words almost soundlessly throughout the day. I put my ear close to his mouth, but I still couldn't make out much of what he was saying. I spoon-fed him some soup and the contents of a fruit cup, but he wasn't very interested in food. Morale-wise, he had reached the lowest point of his hospital stay.

Thankfully, some family visitors came. My brother and sister-in-law spent time with us, and they prayed before they left. My parents later came and my mom prayed. After they left, I prayed over Sam by myself. Sam would later tell me that my mother's prayer stood out the most in his mind.

I left the hospital before freezing rain hit our region that night. Sam spent the rest of night eight all alone. During that stormy night, Sam had a powerful encounter with God. At first, he felt surrounded by warm light. Then a much brighter light appeared that went straight up from the ground in a vertical pillar, about six feet in front of him.

Sam felt a deep peace and a strong assurance of God's love for him. God impressed certain words upon his spirit, which gave him hope he would be healed.

The next morning when I came to the hospital, I met a transformed husband. Animated, cheerful, and energetic, he spoke clearly in a normal voice. His eyes sparkled. He sat up in bed and told me about his experience during the night. His story instantly uplifted my own spirit. I had been praying during the dismal preceding day for the Spirit to directly minister to Sam, because I hadn't been able to help his broken spirit. God heard that prayer.

Sam had encountered a pillar of light without form. I don't think Sam went to heaven (nor does he claim he did). Since Father God and Jesus are enthroned in heaven, this was most likely the Spirit coming to him in the night. I can't explain what happened. You would have to know my husband to recognize how *un*usual this experience was. He had never had an experience like that before. All I know is that Sam went through a profound transformation during night eight in the hospital, touched in some manner by our living God.

Soon after I arrived, Sam was able to get up and walk around the hospital ward for the first time. He needed a walker for a lap or two, but, at one point, he dramatically pushed the walker away, stood up straight and strong, and walked onward with a surreal bounce in his step. One of the ICU doctors walking with me behind Sam said that he couldn't believe what he was seeing. He also remembered how weak, listless, and demoralized Sam had been, just the day before. Literally overnight, God had helped Sam take a *giant* leap forward in his recovery. You can imagine how encouraging this was for all of us.

We can try to encourage ourselves, but we can also ask God to encourage us. Ask for the Spirit to minister to you (or your loved one) in your hour of need. I am pausing to pray that the Spirit *will* minister to you, bringing His light into your dark night.

THE HEALING PROCESS

25

A SEASON OF SUFFERING

I don't fully understand why God might wait weeks, months, years, or even decades before healing someone, or why He permits so much suffering along the way. Suffering can seem cruel and pointless. *Why* does God allow pain and suffering in the lives of His beloved ones? I have learned that God has various reasons for our suffering.

His reasons might lie buried in darkness for a while, waiting to be uncovered. I'll borrow the expression "treasures of darkness" (from Isaiah 45:3) to describe God's purposes in our seasons of suffering. "Treasures of darkness" makes me think of precious jewels concealed within ordinary rocks, secreted in the black depths of the underground world. Have you ever visited the geology section of a natural science museum? I love to visit that area, where cracked-open chunks of rock are on display. Some reveal dazzling shards of white crystal. Others expose exquisite formations of turquoise, lapis lazuli, or malachite. Yet others contain red rubies, blue sapphires, purple amethysts, or green emeralds. The beautiful gemstones shine and sparkle under the display case spotlights.

When we suffer, we can feel trapped in darkness, hemmed in by hard circumstances. Imagine God providing a spiritual shovel and pickaxe, enabling us to dig down through the darkness and strike through the rocky circumstances. Imagine having a divine flashlight, bright enough to illuminate the treasures we find hiding in the darkness of our suffering.

I cannot tell you the specific reason(s) for your suffering. Ask Him for revelation of the treasures He has hidden in your pain. Consider if God has been at work in your health situation in any of the following ways.

Suffering Can Lead Us to Him

Pain, sickness, and suffering can help us to find Him. Surely, *He* is the supreme treasure. After committing my life to Christ at the age of nineteen, I prayed for my dad's salvation on pretty much a daily basis for almost twenty-five years. I concurrently prayed that God would not let my dad die suddenly in a car crash, or by a drop-dead heart attack, until he entered into a relationship with Him. I know that many others prayed for my father along those lines too. One by one, everyone else in my family discovered God through Christ. We all wanted our dad to find Him too.

In my twenty-fifth year of praying those prayers, my father suffered the dual heart attacks that I've told you about, days away from turning sixty-nine years old. My father had those back-to-back heart attacks while on business in Montreal. Thankfully, my mother was with him. From the outset, she prayed extensively, quoting God's words.

After hearing that my dad was in the hospital, I flew to Montreal. I talked with a cardiologist before going to my dad's room. I heard grim news about my dad's heart. The worst news was that his heart might not survive the night. Moments later, I found no comfort in my dad's appearance. Looking pale and tired, he moved weakly.

I realized that I couldn't indulge in casual conversation. I quickly got to the most serious matter. My dad knew the basics about who Christ claimed to be, why He died for us, and the biblical assertion that He rose again. I put the key question to him: Did he want to accept Christ as his Saviour?

To my disappointment, he shook his head sideways and mumbled, "Not tonight." I loved him too much to let the matter rest. I repeated the question, explaining it would only take a few minutes to pray. With surprising strength and firmness in his voice, my dad said: "No, I appreciate you asking me, but not tonight, if you don't mind." The subject was clearly closed. I felt downcast leaving the hospital that night, not knowing if I would see my father again. My mom and I prayed for a while in our hotel room before falling into exhausted sleep.

Over the next days, we kept on praying for Dad's salvation and his healing (as other family members did as well). It was a nerve-wracking time. On doctor's orders, my dad had abruptly stopped smoking. Agitated by the sudden lack of nicotine, he went through cycles of rolling around in his bed until fatigue set in.

The cardiac team wanted to perform an angiogram, followed by angioplasty if possible, and whatever cardiac surgery was warranted by the angiogram results. But first, the hospital had to find litres of extra blood that would match my dad's blood profile. (If heart surgery occurred, my dad might need blood transfusions.) He had been tattooed years before, complicating the search across North American blood banks for matching blood. His own still carried antibodies to some infection he must have sustained back then. Finding suitable blood wasn't easy. Three days went by.

I wrote in my journal: "God is really turning up the heat and tightening the screws. He knows how much pressure He has to bring to bear upon Dad. This is painful to watch, but God is in sovereign control, and His purposes will be accomplished. This is all part of what I have prayed for Dad, that God would use whatever circumstances He has to, to draw Dad to him…"

Finally, a match was found. The requisite litres of blood were flown in. My dad was wheeled on a gurney to a hallway outside an operating room. One of my brothers was with him when a doctor explained the risks of an angiogram, angioplasty, and potential heart surgery. The risks included the possibility of dying on the operating table.

Before my father was taken into the OR, my brother reopened the matter of his salvation, asking him afresh whether he was ready to accept Christ. This time, my dad said yes. They then prayed some version of the sinner's prayer together.

After I heard that great news, I wrote in my journal: "This is an answer to years of prayers, a moment that I have been trusting for all of my adult life."

My whole family thanked God for my dad's monumental decision to accept Christ into his life. We rejoiced that what my dad endured in Montreal brought him to the cross and into an eternal relationship with God. (Twenty years later, my dad is still alive.)

I know many stories of people finding God in the midst of suffering. God used a season of physical pain to draw Brother Andrew to Himself. Prior to becoming a Christian, Andrew served in the Dutch army in Indonesia. In 1949, while in combat, an enemy bullet tore into his ankle. He was medically evacuated and operated on. His doctors weren't certain about his future ability to walk. At best, they surmised, this young man would hobble around with a cane.

Andrew spent months in a field hospital while his ankle slowly healed. Immobile in a leg cast, forced to rest in bed, Andrew grew bored. He started reading the Bible that his mother had packed into his duffle bag before he left Holland. Andrew began to consider whether the Bible was true. He had been resistant to the Christian faith while growing up, even antagonistic sometimes. His resistance began easing as he delved into the Bible with increasing interest.

During his long convalescence, Andrew talked with the kind nuns who ran his hospital ward. He also wrote letters to a young Christian woman in Holland he had a crush on. The quiet hours of private reflection, along with challenging exchanges he had with the nuns and the Dutch woman back home, planted numerous seeds in his spirit.

By his twenty-first birthday, Andrew had recovered enough to take a hospital ship back to Holland. He remained partly lame. Even with the aid of a cane, it hurt to walk. Back on dry land, he tried to forget his troubles through alcohol.

Between nights spent drinking, he attended church. He continued dialogue with the young Dutch woman. He connected with other Christians and began reading his Bible again. Finally, one night in 1950, he prayed alone in his bedroom, turning his life over to God. A year of suffering and searching had brought him to his knees.

Suffering also brought Saul (who later became the apostle Paul) to his knees. Saul, an expert in Jewish law, passionately defended that religion. He persecuted Christians who belonged to the church that emerged in Jerusalem after Jesus ascended. In zealous opposition to that growing church, Saul even murdered believers. Saul began a journey to Damascus, where he planned to persecute more Christians. On his way, "suddenly a light from heaven shone around him" (Acts 9:3) and he heard the voice of Jesus. Saul was blinded by that encounter with the risen Christ (Acts 9:8).

Saul's companions took him to Damascus. He remained blind for three days until Ananias arrived, at the Spirit's beckoning, to pray for him (Acts 9:8–18). Ananias laid hands on Saul (v. 17) and immediately "something like scales fell from his eyes, and he regained his sight. He rose and was baptized" (v. 18).

Why had God afflicted Saul with sudden blindness? Why did God let him suffer for three days and let him wonder if he would ever see again? Perhaps that was necessary for Saul to make the radical 180-degree turn from being a man who murderously persecuted Christians to becoming a dynamic Christian. I suspect that God did a deep work in Saul during the days he was blind, bringing him to the point where he was ready to submit the rest of his life to the Lordship of Christ. After recovering his sight, Saul (Paul) boldly proclaimed Jesus as the Son of God in the synagogues (Acts 9:20).

Suffering for a season has inestimable value if it leads an individual toward a relationship with God. If you're sitting by the bedside of a suffering loved one who has not yet accepted Christ, dare to ask them the questions that will change everything: Can they believe that Christ died for their sins? Will they accept Him into their lives as personal Saviour and Lord? Ask more than once if necessary. Have someone else ask.

Perhaps God has allowed pain and suffering into their lives as a severe mercy, bringing them to a time and place of eternally significant decision making. Having their normal lives disrupted, lying helpless in bed, perhaps even staring death in the face, is what it might take for that loved one to make the decision to seek God through Christ. Their suffering may seem like harsh mercy, but it *is* nonetheless mercy. Pray that your loved one will accept salvation, the greatest mercy of God.

Or perhaps *you* are the one in need of God's mercy. Will *you* choose to ask Jesus to forgive your sins and to become *your* Saviour and Lord? Don't waste the pain and suffering that has brought you to this time and place of reckoning. This is your hour of opportunity. It matters more than anything else on the face of the earth.

When Saul (Paul) was struck blind, he responded to God with a fully receptive heart. Hear the subsequent plea of the apostle Paul to nonbelievers: "... Today, if you hear his voice, do not harden your hearts..." (Hebrews 3:15).

Suffering Can Deepen Our Relationship with God

What if a person is already in a relationship with God? God may use suffering to have that person focus more intently on Him, to better understand who He is, and to tether them more closely to Him. This is what happened to Job.

He "was blameless and upright, one who feared God and turned away from evil" (Job 1:1b). Yet God allowed Job to go through suffering, which included physical pain and sickness, along with discouragement and depression. But eventually Job bowed down to God with increased reverence and deeper appreciation of God as the Almighty Creator and ruler of the universe.

Contemplating his own suffering, Asaph wrote in Psalm 73:26: "My flesh and my heart may fail, but God is the strength of my heart and my portion forever." Although his body and soul were weakening as he penned those words, he chose to turn Godward.

Suffering can deepen our level of commitment to Him. Let's continue the story of Brother Andrew. His ankle pain continued for two more years after the night he turned his life over to God. During that season, Andrew drew even closer to Him. One afternoon during those further years of pain, Andrew prayed a prayer of *full* commitment to God, holding *nothing* back, promising to go wherever God wanted him to go and do whatever God wanted him to do, *despite* the bothersome liability of his crippled ankle. Andrew stood up after he finished that prayer of complete surrender. At first, he felt some sharp pain in his injured ankle. As he began walking home, he realized he could walk better than before. He thought of the Bible story in which ten lepers were healed after they began walking to see the priest, in obedience to what Jesus had instructed. Those men were healed as they walked. So was Andrew. That week, he applied for missionary training, which eventually led to many decades of international ministry.[56]

Are you willing to draw closer to God in your season of suffering? Can you believe that God is spiritually working in a suffering loved one?

Our Suffering Might Bring Someone Else Closer to God

While my husband was in the ICU recovering from his brain bleed, I kept his mobile phone, only letting him use it for short periods so his brain could rest. One morning, he sent a short text to a friend he hadn't seen for a while.

Half an hour later, the friend showed up at the ICU. He had been battling stage-four colon cancer for a few years and had actually just finished some treatment in the same hospital at the time he received Sam's text. He didn't have to go much out of his way to see us.

He stayed and talked with us for a few hours. Up until then, I had never had the courage to come right out and ask our friend if he had accepted Christ into his life. We ended up discussing spiritual matters in depth. We talked about salvation, being confident our sins are forgiven, death, and heaven. Sam and I became assured that our friend was in right standing with God. More importantly, *he* was assured of that. The three of us said to one another, as he was leaving, that we would see each other again, if not in this life then in the next. He was more concerned about my husband's medical condition than his own at that moment.

Within a few months, our friend was gone. Sam later told me that his brain bleed was worth it if it played even a minor part in this friend cementing his relationship with God. Sam had the privilege of praying with our friend just before he died.

That story reminds me of a young man named Jamie who eventually died of cancer. He was the only Christian in his family when he was first diagnosed. His conversations with close family members during his cancer journey led them all to accept Christ. Before Jamie died, he confided to some friends that his suffering had great value in his own eyes, because it had given him much opportunity to speak to his parents and siblings about his faith.

I earlier told you about David Kuo (who once held a senior position in the White House) and his decade-long battle with cancer. He suffered a lot near the end, with severe seizures, mobility issues, anxiety, and the slow collapse of every bodily function. Despite the deterioration of his health, he was able to encourage one of his ICU doctors to read *Mere Christianity*, written by C. S. Lewis.[57] While suffering, he drew others toward God.

I encourage you to notice who is near you during your season of suffering. It may be that God will empower you to make a difference in their lives. I'm not trying to lay a burden on you. I simply want you to see that even a hospital room can be a place of ministry flowing both *to* you and *from* you (as God gives you strength and opportunity).

Suffering Can Help Us Appreciate the Suffering of Christ

When we suffer, we can taste just a little of what Jesus went through on the cross. If we never had to endure physical suffering, we wouldn't be able to appreciate what Jesus experienced for our sakes. In our season of suffering, we can pause to thank Jesus for every moment of suffering He went through for us. We can take the focus off what we're feeling and instead focus on the magnitude of pain He bore.

Our suffering can increase how much we value the love of Jesus and His sacrificial death. If our suffering bonds us more deeply with Christ, then it has accomplished much. Every Easter thereafter can be richer, with an increased measure of adoration, reverence, and gratitude.

Suffering Can Test Our Spiritual Fidelity and Maturity

Suffering can test us just as it tested Job, measuring our faithfulness to God and our true level of spiritual maturity. Satan had challenged God on the issue of Job's uprightness. Satan suggested that Job was blameless only because God had blessed him and put a protective hedge around him. Satan predicted that Job would curse God if God took away the blessings. So God tested Job by allowing him to lose almost everything, from his children to his flocks and herds and his health. Job developed painful sores all over his body, from the crown of his head to the soles of his feet.

How did Job respond? He fell into despair, depression, and inner turmoil. Yet Job said some amazing things while he suffered, such as: "... Naked I came from my mother's womb, and naked I will depart. The Lord gave and the Lord has taken away; may the name of the Lord be praised" (Job 1:21, NIV).

I think Job's finest words are these: "But he [God] knows the way that I take; when he [God] has tried me, I shall come out as gold. My foot has held fast to his steps; I have kept his way and have not turned aside" (Job 23:10–11).

God blessed Job after his long season of suffering. He gave Job twice as much as he had before (Job 42:10). "The Lord blessed the latter part of Job's life more than the former part" (Job 42:12a, NIV). Job died when he was "an old man and full of years" (Job 42:17, NIV).

Suffering exposes our innermost self. Can we resolve, like Job, to come through the fiery furnace of our affliction as purified gold? Can we remain faithful to God throughout our period of suffering? How will *we* react when God tests us? A season of suffering will show us the answer to those questions.

Suffering Can Lead to Necessary Correction

Maybe we won't do so well in the test of our faithfulness and maturity. A season of suffering can produce necessary spiritual correction. A psalmist wrote: "I shall not die, but I shall live, and recount the deeds of the Lord. The Lord has disciplined me severely, but he has not given me over to death" (Psalm 118:17–18). The first verse can roll off of our lips easily. The second verse is more disturbing. There must have been reasons that the Lord disciplined this psalmist, allowing him to suffer almost to the point of death. The tone of the two verses suggests that both God and the psalmist considered the discipline of suffering necessary.

Suffering can expose sin. The Lord spoke to rebellious Israel and Judah:

> *For thus says the Lord: Your hurt is incurable, and your wound is*
> *grievous. There is none to uphold your cause, no medicine for your*
> *wound, no healing for you... I have dealt you the blow of an enemy,*
> *the punishment of a merciless foe, because your guilt is great,*
> *because your sins are flagrant... I have done these things to you.*
> Jeremiah 30:12–15

But in verse 17 of the same chapter, we see God's mercy and grace: "... I will restore health to you, and your wounds I will heal, declares the Lord..." God planned to *later* restore His people, but first He would let suffering chasten and correct them.

Perhaps there are times when you, as a parent, have had to exercise tough love. If you have a teenager who recklessly drinks, breaks curfew, and maybe even breaks the law, you have to discipline that teenager *because* you love them. You might ground them or refuse to post bail to get them out of jail if they have been in trouble repeatedly. God might also discipline us with some tough love, if it's warranted.

Suffering Can Produce Dependence on God

When times are easy, we might slip into self-sufficiency. Suffering often compels us to depend on God. In her book *Out of Darkness*, Stormie Omartian described the excruciating abdominal pain she endured because of a ruptured appendix that wasn't diagnosed quickly. Toxic fluid spread through her abdomen. When the problem was finally diagnosed, she had to undergo emergency surgery. The surgeons couldn't clean out all of the toxins. They had to leave an eighteen-inch open incision to allow the poison to be mechanically suctioned out. Stormie was unable to eat or drink for many days. Morphine, antibiotics, and fluids were pumped into her intravenously. The long surgical wound remained open for five months, during which she required further surgery to remove her gallbladder.

Her physical suffering didn't end there. For fifteen years, she suffered long-term consequences of the toxins that had assaulted her internal organs and body systems. She developed new health issues. She dealt with high cholesterol, osteoporosis, hormonal imbalance, a weakened immune system, migraine headaches, and digestive issues.

Stormie stated that her long years of medical struggles caused her to become totally dependent on God, more than she had ever been. She realized afresh that her life was completely in God's hands. She had to rely on His goodness, grace, provision, and healing power. God spared her life and, over time, has resolved many of the residual consequences of the delayed diagnosis.[58]

Suffering Can Forge Stronger Character

The apostle Paul wrote:

Through him [the Lord Jesus Christ] we have also obtained access
by faith into this grace in which we stand, and we rejoice in hope
of the glory of God. Not only that, but we rejoice in our sufferings,
knowing that suffering produces endurance, and endurance
produces character, and character produces hope…

Romans 5:2–4

Suffering can be a catalyst for character growth. Suffering can strengthen us. We can become unshakably strong, ready to handle any of life's challenges, if we allow God to work in us. We can develop a solid steel core in the furnace of affliction. We can learn that all things are bearable as we let Him impart His strength to us.

Suffering can also force us to deal with negative character qualities, such as our pride. Sickness and weakness can be incredibly humbling. Any grown person who has had to wear a diaper can attest to that, as can any adult who has been bathed, dressed, or fed by others. If suffering can turn our haughtiness into humility, we will be better people as a result.

Suffering Can Produce Compassion

Suffering can create more empathy and compassion in us. We can learn how to comfort others with the comfort that we have received (from God and others) in our season of suffering. After we've experienced pain ourselves, we're usually more sensitive to the pain of others.

Hospital visits occasionally trigger memories of my childhood hospitalizations. I remember the fatigue; the aches and pains; and the feelings of self-pity, fear, and loneliness. I recall eating meal after not-so-tasty meal while bed-trapped, staring out the window, wishing I could go home, dreaming of returning to my normal world, wondering if I ever would. I now thank God for my own days in a hospital bed. I know that any measure of compassion I show others has its roots in the measure of suffering I have endured (which is nowhere near the suffering of many).

Sometimes I walk past the hospital I stayed in. I know the exact window I used to look out of during my longest admission. It's the second one from the south end on the fifth floor. It overlooks a busy boulevard. On occasion, I stand on the boulevard and look up at my old window, wondering who is in the bed on the other side of it. I pause to pray for whoever is occupying that bed that day.

Toronto's leading hospitals line that same street. They offer help to cancer patients, cardiac patients, sick children, and others. I have visited family members and friends when they've been patients in those hospitals. When I walk down the length of that street, I take a moment to pray for all of the patients in all of the hospitals located there.

Cars and pedestrians rush by. I wonder: If those passers-by have never suffered in those hospitals, do they give them a moment's thought as they whiz by? Probably not. Compassion flows easiest out of the heart that has suffered much and shared in the sufferings of others. Purpose to let your suffering form more compassion in your heart.

Suffering Can Knit People Together

Colossians 2:2 talks about hearts "being knit together in love." That verse has come to mind during healing journeys. I have special memories of times spent with loved ones in the hospital and later at home as they (or I) recovered more. Suffering can strengthen the bonds in a marriage or a family, drawing people closer.

Sometime after Stormie's ruptured appendix, her husband was diagnosed with non-Hodgkin's lymphoma, a type of cancer. Stormie sat with him during eight-hour-long chemotherapy infusions. Those shared experiences blessed their relationship. They knew that this kind of crisis could blow their marriage apart or bond them together in love and commitment. They *chose* to let the situation bring them closer together.[59]

Suffering might bring reconciliation between family members or friends who have grown distant. When a spouse or parent is sick, they might apologize and request forgiveness for hurts they have caused.

This happened to a lawyer I knew after he was diagnosed with advanced cancer. He apologized to his ex-wife for leaving their marriage and asked her to forgive him. She did. Wounds were healed in both of them. I saw the adult children of another friend (also diagnosed with terminal cancer) make peace with one another, ending a period of tension and estrangement. Suffering has a way of bringing members of a church congregation together. I've seen this in my own church when various members have been gravely ill.

Suffering Can Improve Our Perspective

After we've recovered from an injury, illness, or surgery, we might see the world in a whole new light. Many cancer patients say that after they've gone through surgery, radiation, and chemotherapy for months or years, normal daily problems seem miniscule. What does it matter if a child spills their milk? What's the big deal if a car door gets scratched? A cancer survivor might enjoy ordinary days, full of ordinary problems, better than many others. They might see their blessings more clearly. Suffering can make us grateful for what once seemed routine, even tedious.

Author Kay Warren, wife of megachurch pastor Rick Warren, has written about the many treasures she discovered in the darkness of suffering. In 2003, she was diagnosed with breast cancer. Less than two years later, she was diagnosed with melanoma. As a result of her cancer journeys, she learned how precious every single day is, how fragile life is. This fresh perspective gave her increased passion for making every day count.

Kay was determined to learn new lessons when three further crises happened in 2008: A grandson born premature nearly died; that baby's mother, who also nearly died, required three surgeries because of a brain tumour and subsequent brain complications; and a son was hospitalized for serious mental illness. During that tumultuous year, Kay changed her perspective on suffering. It was no longer her enemy.

She decided to embrace suffering and look for what God was trying to teach her.[60]

Sickness and Suffering Can Provide Forced Rest

Sickness can sometimes provide us with much-needed rest on many levels. A friend took time off work during treatment for breast cancer. Although her treatment wasn't easy, she enjoyed a long rest from her career and other responsibilities. She had been exhausted and on over-drive before her cancer diagnosis. She hadn't been taking care of her health and had felt run down. Her necessary period of rest allowed her to sleep in some days, put her feet up on the couch many afternoons, linger over cups of tea, read books she had been wanting to read, and catch up with old friends. She had ample time to pray and read the Bible. She didn't just get physical rest. She received deep spiritual, mental, and emotional rest. In some ways, even during treatment, she felt better than she'd felt in a long time.

I've had many people tell me that they too experienced multi-faceted rest during time away from regular routines for treatment, rehabilitation, and recovery.

The Suffering of One Might Alleviate the Suffering of Others

The physical suffering of one person can shine a bright light on the suffering of others. This occurred in the life of an American physician, Dr. Kent Brantly. I had the privilege of meeting Dr. Brantly when he spoke at Canada's National Prayer Breakfast.

Dr. Brantly and his wife, with two children in tow, began serving as medical missionaries in Liberia, West Africa, in 2013, with a Christian organization called World Medical Mission (the medical arm of Samaritan's Purse). Dr. Brantly worked at the ELWA Hospital, a place I can visualize. My husband, Sam, served as a short-term doctor there on two occasions, in 1980 and 1985, bringing me along the second time.

An Ebola outbreak struck West Africa in spring 2014. Ebola is one of the world's most dreaded deadly viruses. At the time, there was no medical cure. The outbreak quickly spread from where it originated, in Guinea, to the nearby countries of Sierra Leone and Liberia. It soon became the worst known outbreak of the disease in the world's history.

Organizations such as Doctors Without Borders and World Medical Mission worked with local health authorities. As the crisis spread, they asked for help from the United Nations, the World Health Organization, and other international medical contacts. Despite urgent requests, the frontline doctors received little support. They worked long hours under difficult, dangerous circumstances.

Dr. Brantly became the director of the Ebola Center at ELWA Hospital, which housed about fifty beds. The ELWA chapel was quickly converted into an isolation unit. Although Dr. Brantly and his team took all possible precautions, they constantly risked becoming infected by the highly contagious virus. They wore heavy protective gear, including head coverings, gloves, and boots, which tortured them in the tropical heat. Changing outfits several times daily, they kept running low on the gear.

Ebola robs patients of their control over their bodily functions. Diapers and sheets had to be continually changed. Patients writhed and groaned in pain.

Within a few months, thousands of Liberians were stricken with the disease, and around half of them died. Dr. Brantly stood by the beds of many dying patients, daring to hold their hands. He may not have physically saved every life, but I trust that many souls were saved because of his brave, compassionate service.

Dr. Brantly fell prey to the vicious virus and grew very sick in summer 2014. He eventually flew on an emergency medevac flight to Atlanta, Georgia, where Emory University Hospital placed him in an isolation unit. The international press reported his arrival and subsequent medical progress. Ebola had come to America. It was front-page news. The world watched and waited. Even with the best possible medical care, no one could guarantee that Dr. Brantly would survive.

His life truly rested in God's hands. Along with countless other Christians, I prayed for Dr. Brantly. Thankfully, Dr. Brantly lived through his ordeal. He would later publicly proclaim that God had delivered him.

Some might question why God would allow such a courageous, self-sacrificing doctor to suffer so much for so long instead of leaving him to serve on the frontlines. Although I don't presume to know God's reasons, it seems to me that Dr. Brantly's battle with Ebola brought much-needed publicity and a sense of urgency to the worsening situation in West Africa. It's one thing to read about people dying halfway around the world. It's quite another to recognize how quickly the virus could arrive on a plane to any North American city. Less than a week after Dr. Brantly arrived in Atlanta, the U.S. Congress began a hearing on the Ebola crisis. The United Nations and the World Health Organization began to take the escalating Ebola outbreak much more seriously. Governments of many nations committed more money, medical help, and technical personnel to the cause.

If Dr. Brantly had remained healthy in Liberia, he could have saved some further lives. Because he personally fought the life-threatening illness, an exponentially greater number of lives were likely saved because of the media attention his Ebola fight commanded. God used Dr. Brantly's weeks of suffering to generate a new influx of resources from around the world. The spread of the virus was eventually curbed.

Suffering Can Help Us to Finish Well

Suffering can lead us to appropriately number our days. It might force us to get our affairs in order. It might be the push we need to write a will, give things away, sell property, and otherwise simplify our estate for the sake of our executors and heirs. In contrast, those who die suddenly don't always leave their estate in optimal shape.

Suffering can be the harbinger of death. It poses big questions. What do we want to say or do before we die? Do we want to talk to certain people about Christ? Do we want to tell them we love them?

Do we want to say we're sorry for something? Do we want to say our final goodbyes? End-of-life suffering can offer such opportunities.

The Secular World Doesn't Value Suffering

Some Western nations have legalized euthanasia or medically assisted death. (Euthanasia occurs when the doctor directly causes the death. In medically assisted death jurisdictions, the doctor provides the legal means, such as lethal drugs, which the patient uses to cause their own death.) Those in favour of right-to-die laws argue that they allow for a compassionate end to pain. Those proponents see no value in suffering. Euthanasia or medically assisted death has been legalized in Belgium, Holland, Switzerland, some American states, and now Canada.

There's an unspoken reason that many governments permit death on demand. Such unnatural deaths can save government health departments (and/or insurance companies) gazillions of dollars. I heard of one study that concluded that half of the average person's medical bills are racked up in the last six months of their life. If cancer patients, for example, end their lives early, imagine all the money that could be saved by government and insurance providers. Such providers know that one lethal dose of a drug is much cheaper than extended medical care. Cold, hard economics may be the main driver behind laws that allow death on demand. All the talk about a compassionate, dignified end to suffering makes for a great marketing pitch to the public, masking the economic rationale. We can expect the scope of death on demand laws to broaden as the Baby Boomers age. Their declining health will place unprecedented strain on the budgets of health systems and insurance providers in the Western world.

God has allowed seasons of pain and suffering for the many good reasons we have discussed. A premature end to suffering could thwart such purposes, including the most important purposes of drawing individuals into relationship (or deeper relationship) with God. What if the person has not yet made their peace with God? Their premature death might shorten their suffering in this life but prolong their eternal suffering (which will have no end).

Not Wasting Our Suffering

It is possible to waste our suffering. My subtitles suggest that suffering *can* be a catalyst for certain things to happen. Suffering does not *automatically* lead to all of the results I've listed. We have to *choose* what suffering will produce in us. Like Kay Warren, we can embrace our pain and discover many of its purposes as we wait upon our healing. Suffering can transform us into better people, if we let it. Whether we're personally suffering or vicariously suffering alongside an ailing loved one, we can permit suffering to perform good work within us. Ask God what He is trying to accomplish with your suffering. Resolve, like Job, to come forth as gold on the other side of it.

The Suffering *Will* End

We can rejoice in the reality that *all* suffering will one day come to an end, if not in this life then in the next. For some, the release from suffering will come only at death. If loved ones have died in right relationship with God, we can rejoice that their season of suffering has passed, and they have crossed over to a place where they will never suffer again.

26

GOD'S TIMING

We cannot control the timing of our healing. We can *influence* the timing of our healing, to some extent, by taking steps such as praying and seeking medical help. Ultimately, God decides the matter.

When Jesus heard that his dear friend Lazarus was sick, He didn't go to him immediately. Instead, He waited for a few days. Jesus wasn't being callous or indifferent to the sickness of His friend. According to John, Jesus loved Lazarus and his sisters. Jesus delayed coming to see Lazarus for a good reason.

By the time Jesus arrived at Lazarus' town, His friend had been buried for four days. Jesus glorified God by raising Lazarus from the dead. Jesus knew all along what was going to happen. He was deliberate in His timing.

Restoration might come sooner than we expect, or it might come much later.

Healing might occur as a singular event, in a moment in time, or, more likely, it will come as a *process* over time. Sometimes God heals quickly, in a day or two. Other times, He heals over weeks, months, or years. God determines the timetable.

Instant or Almost-Instant Healing

Is there really such a thing as instant healing? Many people seem to have been instantly healed in the Bible, their stories taking place in a particular moment in time. We discussed in an earlier chapter that most New Testament healings probably had a backstory of prayer, faith, and pressing in. The disappearance of tangible symptoms, however, seemed to occur suddenly when a sick person encountered Jesus. When someone appears to be healed quickly, we call this a miracle. Natural healing usually takes time. Sudden healing has a supernatural quality to it.

Personally, I see all healing as having a miraculous dimension. I like what Albert Einstein said: "There are only two ways to live your life. One is as though nothing is a miracle. The other is as if everything is." Isn't the way our body heals a skin cut quite amazing? Aren't modern medical treatments miracles of sorts?

Yet I must concede that the Bible does seem to portray a miracle as something quite out of the ordinary. Then and now, such moment-in-time miracles point people to the kingdom of God breaking into their situations. God's glory seems to be more manifest after an instant healing than after a slow healing that appears to arise from the body's inherent systems and processes, or by medical means (although God is, of course, *very* involved in natural and medical processes). Jesus performed many moment-in-time miracles. The disciples and apostles also performed miraculous healings, by God's power, after Jesus left this earth.

Billy Graham believed that many people have been miraculously healed in recent times. While he didn't understand why God heals some people and not others, he admitted that miraculous healings still happen.[61] Many other modern Christians hold the same belief.

I hear of wonders happening all over the world today, proving that God cares just as much about drawing people to Him today as He did about those who lived in the time of Jesus. Many stories come from other continents where hearts and minds aren't so skeptical about supernatural occurrences.

New Testament professor and author Craig S. Keener travelled to the Congo, where his wife's family lived. He heard seven eyewitness accounts of people being healed, even after they appeared to have died. His mother-in-law, for example, told him the story of how one of her daughters was bitten by a snake when she was a child. The little girl stopped breathing. No medical help could be sought locally, so Keener's mother-in-law carried her daughter to another village where an evangelist prayed for her. The little child started to breathe again (after three hours of *not* breathing). If you're wondering whether the child sustained brain damage during those three hours without oxygen, I can tell you this: The child grew up to obtain a master's degree.[62] If you go searching for such stories, you will find them.

If you want a miracle, approach God with faith. Remind Him of the many moment-in-time miracles that Jesus and His followers performed back in biblical times, and of the many miracles that continue to occur in our times. Ask for your miracle, but then leave the outcome in His hands. God will decide whether you're spontaneously healed or healed over some period of time.

I've never been healed instantly, but I have been healed, on several occasions, quite rapidly. Let me tell you about four occasions of almost-instant healing, which all occurred after I had attended a church service where my healing was prayed for.

Years ago, after suffering significant and sustained pain in one molar, I consulted my dentist. He sent my X-rays to a dental specialist. Soon after, I was told my tooth had some nerve damage and would require a root canal procedure. Before the root canal surgical appointment, I went to a church healing service, seeking prayer for a family member with a problem more serious than my aching tooth. Moments after my late arrival, the speaker asked anyone who needed dental healing to stand up. I did so, marvelling that this was happening. The speaker prayed for everyone standing. In the quietness of my own heart, I prayed in agreement with him. I didn't feel anything happen during or after the prayer time. My tooth still ached.

When I woke up the next morning, the toothache was gone. It didn't come back. I never did have a root canal on that tooth. More than eighteen years have passed. Then and now, I give glory to God for that rapid, dentally inexplicable healing.

I once attended a similar kind of healing service in Buffalo, New York. A well-known evangelist presided. In India, I had recently battled malaria. (I've already shared some of this story.) With medication, the malaria had cleared up. I seemed fine until my hair started falling out back in Canada. For weeks, I lost strands at a much faster rate than normal. After two discouraging prognoses from medical specialists, I was desperate enough to heed my mom's suggestion to attend the healing service in Buffalo.

At the service, fear and faith jostled for supremacy. I listened to the evangelist's talk and to his prayer for the whole crowd. Too many people were in attendance for a healing line to form, so no one prayed personally for my need.

Nothing tangible happened that night or in the first few days following the service. One morning, however, less than a week later, everything changed quite suddenly. When brushing my hair, I noticed that barely any hair was collecting in the brush. The next time I washed my hair, only a *few* strands had to be washed down the drain. The hair loss stopped remarkably quickly, and new hair grew in with astounding speed. Then and now, I give glory to God for that sudden turnaround.

My third experience with almost-instant healing occurred soon after I attended a special healing service at yet another church. I was there to pray for a loved one. The healing evangelist who conducted the meeting was a young fellow, a bit of a firecracker, with spiky, bleached hair. He only had an elementary school education, yet he seemed to know the Bible well. He quoted many long passages of scripture from memory. That night, he also purported to operate in the gifts of knowledge, prophecy, and healing. I wasn't sure what to make of him.

In the midst of him calling out words of knowledge about various individuals, he stated that a woman in the room had been experiencing pain on the right side of her neck, radiating down her shoulder, and that sometimes when she used her right arm, the resulting pain felt as if a muscle extending down her neck was "ripping." Those last words caught my attention. That muscle-ripping reference mimicked how I had described a recurring tennis injury to my husband. Such muscle pain had flared up several times over the previous year while playing tennis. I was experiencing pain in my neck and right shoulder that night.

The evangelist asked the described woman to come forward. No one got up. I *knew* that he was referring to me. I sensed that God was asking me to step out in faith, so I did. I went to the front of the room, and the unorthodox young man prayed for me.

I had never met that speaker before. He lived on the other side of the country. The service was being held in a church I'd never attended. I'd decided to come to the service at the last moment, so it wasn't possible that anyone had tipped him off about me. It seemed to me that God had given him divine knowledge about my injury.

I didn't feel any different when I sat down. I woke up the next morning, however, with all pain in my neck and shoulder gone. That distinctive pain never came back, even though I continued to play tennis for years. Then and now, I give glory to God for that very rapid, unusual healing.

My fourth (and most recent) almost-instant healing took place in a Texas megachurch. I arrived at the Sunday service with blister-like sores on both hands. I had been plagued with that irritating skin condition off and on for a year. My dermatologist had prescribed a cream that helped to gradually heal the skin condition each time it flared up, but it was hard to keep the cream on my hands. I often washed my hands during the day in the course of activities such as gardening and food preparation.

During the service, congregants were invited to come forward for prayer for healing. Senior church members waited at the front, intending to pray for each one personally. Too many people ahead of me poured into the aisles. The senior pastor, knowing not everyone could be prayed for individually, prayed generally for the rest of us.

Assenting in my heart to the powerful words of the pastor, I specifically asked God to heal my pain-prickled hands.

I'd learned from experience not to be disappointed if I didn't feel immediate results. The numerous eruptions on my hands bothered me the rest of that day, even more than usual, because of the scorching Texas heat and heavy humidity.

I woke up the next morning with every blister gone and the skin of both palms perfectly normal. The sores have never returned in the many years since that service.

I don't believe any of those experiences were coincidences. I don't believe that I just happened to feel better within day(s) after each church service. I think we're all smart enough to recognize when physical healing has occurred with unnatural, abnormal, sudden speed.

When He wants to, God can make symptoms disappear the way that water evaporates on a hot day, vanishing into thin air.

Gradual Healing

Usually, we're *gradually* healed from most maladies, including coughs, colds, flus, cuts, bruises, and broken bones. God has programmed our bodies to heal slowly and naturally in most cases. This is the most common kind of healing.

Let's not belittle gradual, natural healing. It's a form of healing, and it comes from the gracious hand of God who made our bodies the way He did. After we become Christians, our spiritual transformation is gradual. So is our mental and emotional transformation. Why do we expect physical healing to always be instant or speedy?

I've told you about the childhood disease I struggled with. My healing process took months (with respect to some symptoms) and years (with respect to others). I had to be healed from both the disease and the effects of the prescribed medication.

Brother Andrew waited eighteen years to be healed of his painful back condition.

Isaac prayed for his wife, Rebekah, to bear children. After twenty years of infertility, she conceived and delivered twin boys, Jacob and Esau (Genesis 25:20–26).

My mom had a kidney disease called nephritis when she was thirteen years old. For a whole year, she stayed home from school and was often confined to her bed. She read a lot of books and played the piano. She recalls often kneeling at the piano bench in the living room during that time, asking God for healing. She wasn't supposed to go outside, but sometimes she would sneak downstairs in the middle of the night. She'd open the back door to breathe in the fresh air and would look up to the stars and pray for healing. After one full year, she was healed and has lived on for more than seven decades without any recurrence of nephritis. (She now believes she would have been healed faster had she known then what God's Word says about healing.)

As we pray for healing, we can ask ourselves: has there been *any* improvement over time? Is the pain lessening? Does a limb have greater range of motion? Is inflammation subsiding? Can we stop taking certain medications? Such improvements, however gradual, should be cause for praise and gratitude. They can provide sustenance for ongoing faith, hope, and patience.

Some healing is so subtle and gradual, we don't even notice it happening. For years, my mom was supposed to wear glasses while driving. At the age of eighty, provincial law decreed that she had to have her vision tested. She was delighted when a government clerk told her that she no longer required driving glasses. Her distance vision had improved to the point of being within normal range.

I had an interesting experience with my own eyes. When I was in my early forties, an eye specialist told me that I had a small cataract growing in one eye. He predicted that I would need cataract surgery by the age of fifty. Foolishly, I didn't get my eyes examined again for years. When I finally had them re-examined in my mid-fifties, the cataract was gone. I hadn't noticed any change in my vision. Just like disease can slowly grow in our body without us being aware of it for a while, healing can gradually occur in our bodies without us detecting the process.

Progressive Healing

Mark 8:22–25 tells the story of a blind man who was healed in progressive stages. Jesus touched his eyes and, at first, the blind man received partial vision. He told Jesus that people looked like trees walking around. Jesus touched him again, and then his vision was fully restored. Jesus could have healed him completely with His first touch. I believe this story happened to show us that we, too, can be healed in progressive stages. After we're partially healed, we can ask for greater healing.

Healing That Has Not Fully Happened Yet

Many people say that they have prayed for healing and it *never* happened. Why not say they have not been healed *yet*? *Yet* implies faith and hope that God *will* heal them some day.

I have some physical needs that I've prayed about but that still persist. I'm still waiting for God to heal me in those areas. I choose to say God hasn't healed me *yet*. I trust that, one day, He will. Why abandon faith and hope? Why give up? Why expect God to cooperate with *our* preferred timetable and, when He doesn't, assume He doesn't care and won't act? It can take as much emotional energy to *press hope down* as it does to *lift it up*.

We should consider remission, or the successful management of chronic illness to the point where we have reasonable quality of life, as forms of substantial healing. My father, for example, was diagnosed with a type of lymphoma cancer at the age of eighty-four. He underwent chemotherapy for a few years and has been in steady remission since then. He functions quite well for his age. While we cannot say he's been completely healed, he has certainly been substantially healed.

Healing in Eternity

We've already talked about receiving perfect restoration in the next life. We discussed Hebrews 11. That profound passage explains much, while leaving some questions unanswered. *Many* biblical heroes of faith received what God had promised them in *this* life, but others had to wait for promises to be fulfilled in the next life. The people listed in Hebrews 11 had faith about a wide range of matters, not necessarily health issues, although we know that some "were made strong out of weakness" (Hebrews 11:34). Faith can apply to all areas of our lives, including healing.

Hebrews 11:13 refers to people who died before promises were fulfilled: "These all died in faith, *not* having received the things promised, but having seen them and greeted them from afar..." Hebrews 11:39 refers again to those who "... though commended through their faith, did not receive what was promised..." Hebrews 11:13–16 describe how they were "strangers" and "exiles" on earth that sought the "better country" of heaven. They can now, in heaven, *fully* see how God fulfilled His promises.

The timeline of a Christian's life is an unbroken *continuum* from *this* life into eternity. Let's stop drawing a solid line between this life and the next.

Hebrews 11:1 states: "Now faith is the assurance of things hoped for, the conviction of things not seen." By faith, we can believe certain things and be assured of them, even if we don't get to see them in this lifetime. Who are we to limit the fulfillment of God's promises to the here-and-now?

I don't pretend to fully understand Hebrews 11. It contains great mystery. I don't understand why some people receive what is promised in this life, and others have to wait until the next. But I must accept this reality to the degree that I can understand it. I will hope for answers to my prayers to materialize in my lifetime, but if I'm one of those who leave this earth with some prayers still unanswered, don't feel sad for me. I believe there's a better life ahead. In my eternal home, I shall be able to see all answers to all good prayers, even if they come to pass after my earthly pilgrimage.

The thought of death shouldn't disturb us. As soon as we die, we shall instantly rise in spirit to be with Father God and Jesus the risen Son. We know this because of the conversation Jesus had with the thief who was nailed to a cross beside Him. The thief implored: "Jesus, remember me when you come into your kingdom" (Luke 23:42). Jesus responded: "Truly, I say to you, today you will be with me in paradise" (v. 43).

When we first go to heaven, we'll be there as spiritual beings but will not yet exist in bodily form. We know this from some passages written by the apostle Paul:

> *... we do not lose heart. Though our outer self is wasting away,*
> *our inner self is being renewed day by day. For this light momen-*
> *tary affliction is preparing for us an eternal weight of glory beyond*
> *all comparison, as we look not to the things that are seen but to the*
> *things that are unseen. For the things that are seen are transient,*
> *but the things that are unseen are eternal... We know that while*
> *we are at home in the body we are away from the Lord... we would*
> *rather be away from the body and at home with the Lord.*
>
> 2 Corinthians 4:16b–18; 5:6b, 8

In 1 Corinthians 15:42–44, Paul further disclosed:

> *So is it with the resurrection of the dead. What is sown [on earth]*
> *is perishable; what is raised is imperishable. It is sown in dishonor;*
> *it is raised in glory. It is sown in weakness; it is raised in power.*
> *It is sown a natural body; it is raised a spiritual body. If there is a*
> *natural body, there is also a spiritual body.*

Our *physical* bodies will be resurrected later, at the Second Coming of Christ (1 Thessalonians 4:14–17). Paul elaborates on that *bodily* resurrection in 1 Corinthians 15:51–53:

Behold! I tell you a mystery. We shall not all sleep, but we shall all be changed, in a moment, in the twinkling of an eye, at the last trumpet. For the trumpet will sound, and the dead will be raised imperishable, and we shall be changed. For this perishable body must put on the imperishable, and this mortal body must put on immortality.

When our physical bodies are raised at the time Christ returns, they will become permanent and indestructible. All in God's good timing…

27

OBSTACLES

Mark 1:32–34 describes a scene in which all of the sick people in a town came to Jesus, but not all were healed: "That evening… the people brought to Jesus *all* the sick… The whole town gathered… and Jesus healed *many* who had various diseases" (NIV).

This story differs from some other stories in which Jesus healed everyone who came to Him. Why didn't He heal every person in the Mark 1:32–34 story? We will never know what His reasons were in that situation, but other verses reveal *some* of the reasons that God doesn't heal everyone.

We might pray for "breakthrough" in the illness we're concerned about. The concept of breakthrough assumes that there's some sort of obstacle blocking the healing, like icebergs impeding movement in a shipping channel. Here are some potential obstacles that might be standing in the way of us receiving healing. It's up to us to remove such obstacles.

A Theology of Unbelief

Unbelief hinders the work of God. Jesus did not "do many mighty works there [in Nazareth], because of their unbelief" (Matthew 13:58).

The New Testament provides many statements to the effect that we must *believe* before we receive something; we won't likely receive if we don't believe (see, for example, James 1:6–8).

You might recall that prayer for healing, common in the first three centuries after Christ ascended, became watered down over the next sixteen centuries. Unbelief regarding the access of ordinary Christians to God's healing power became rampant. Some theologians taught that divine healing (initiated by believers) ended with the first apostles or, at the latest, with the closing of the canon of scripture about four centuries later. God supposedly gave a special outpouring of the healing gift during that limited timeframe to catalyze the growth of the early church. Surely the church needs to be catalyzed in *this* age, too! Unbelief regarding our access to God's healing power remains quite widespread in today's church. Paul prophesied that many people in the last days who *appear* on the surface to be godly would *deny the power* of godliness (2 Timothy 3:5).

Unbelief is self-perpetuating. A person (or a church) that believes that God doesn't heal in response to prayer won't pray for healing. (If they do pray, it might be at the last moment, as an act of desperation.) It's no surprise that persons in such congregations rarely receive healing. The culture of unbelief gets reinforced. Individual faith becomes difficult to cultivate. Parishioner after parishioner might suffer and die. The theology of unbelief gets further strengthened with each death. An entire church can become a Nazareth-like community of unbelief.

It's only human to have *some* measure of unbelief. Mark 9:17–29 talks about a man who brought his son to Jesus for healing, telling Him that a spirit often seized his son, muted him, and threw him down on the ground. His son would then become rigid, grind his teeth, and foam at the mouth. His son had even fallen into fire or water during the course of a seizure. Jesus told the father: "… All things are possible for one who believes" (Mark 9:23). The father responded: "I believe; help my unbelief!" (v. 24). We don't know why the man had some unbelief. He'd brought his son to the disciples, asking them to heal the boy. The disciples tried to heal him but could not. Perhaps that triggered his unbelief.

Jesus, moved by the man's request for help overcoming his unbelief, healed the man's son. I imagine that removed all unbelief. Bring any unbelief you might have to Jesus. He wants to help you dispel it.

If you're surrounded by people who don't believe that access to God's healing power is still available today, consider finding support elsewhere. A church community that actively teaches about healing will help your own faith to grow. You'll also receive the benefit of corporate faith being exercised on your behalf.

An Attitude of Defeat

While seeking healing, we might face spiritual opposition. The faint of heart might let opposition defeat them. Many opposed Jesus when He healed the sick. The religious authorities, threatened by (and perhaps jealous of) the growing popularity of Jesus, conspired against Him. Jesus kept on healing despite the opposition. Even the cross didn't defeat Him. On the cross, He won victory over sin, disease, and death.

After Jesus ascended, His disciples carried on His healing work. Peter and John, for example, publicly healed a crippled man in the name of Jesus (Acts 4). The two disciples were then promptly arrested, put into custody, and hauled in front of the Jewish leaders. The religious leaders knew they couldn't deny the healing, but they didn't want an encore. So those leaders tried to intimidate Peter and John, warning them not to speak again in the name of Jesus. Peter and John continued to teach and to heal the sick in the name of Jesus. They didn't allow opposition to stop their efforts.

If Jesus and His followers faced opposition, hostility, and persecution for healing the sick, then we, too, can expect some measure of the same treatment along the way. If we openly seek God's healing power long enough (for our own selves or others), we will likely encounter some spiritual resistance.

Don't crumble when opposition comes. Don't give in to theological bullying. Don't waste energy on heated intellectual debate. Don't allow yourself to be defeated by others or by the enemy of your soul.

Believing It's Wrong to Ask for Healing

Some people believe it's wrong to ask for healing. They point to Mark 8:11–12. In that passage, some men demanded that Jesus show them a miraculous sign. Jesus refused. Why? He had already performed miraculous healings all over Israel. I submit that Jesus didn't want to perform miracles for the men in the Mark 8 story because they were *demanding* miracles as a sign, *wanting proof* of who He was—*testing* Him.

In contrast to the situation described in Mark 8:11–12, Jesus performed wonderful healings on many other occasions for those who *acknowledged* who He was and had *faith* in Him and who came to Him *humbly presenting* their need. Such people didn't care about Jesus proving anything. They were already convinced that He had the power of God working in Him. Many already believed in Him as the Son of God.

We can ask God for healing not because we demand a sign of who He is, but simply because we need healing. It's not selfish to ask for healing. Healing will bring glory to God and encourage others.

Expecting God to Do Everything

God's healing power doesn't usually come down without us having to do something. In His Word, God has asked us to do many things, such as praying, exercising our faith, and taking good care of our bodies. We must do our part as best we can before we expect Him to do His part in the healing process. Seeking healing with a lazy spirit will not likely avail much.

Lack of True Desire

Some people don't want to get well. Jesus asked a lame man (who had not been able to walk for thirty-eight years) whether he *wanted* to get well (John 5:6). Jesus knew that some people prefer to hold on to their infirmity.

There are "benefits" to remaining sick. Illness can provide: attention, the hope that family and friends might visit or call more often, an excuse for not working or achieving anything, sympathy, medical insurance payments or financial gain from a legal claim, and many other "rewards."

In the John 5 story, Jesus made the lame man *decide* whether or not he wanted to get well. Jesus told the man to pick up his mat and begin walking (v. 8). The man faced a choice. He could stay lying down and remain infirm or he could demonstrate his desire to get well by obeying Jesus. The lame man must have been sick of being sick. He picked up his mat and started walking, and "at once the man was healed" (v. 9).

Not everyone makes that quality choice. Loved ones and medical personnel may try to help them get better, but they obstinately undermine such help. They don't take their medications. They refuse the reasonable option of surgery. They don't eat well, even though they know better and have the resources to do so. They don't get up off the couch to exercise, even when their doctor has told them they need to. Their actions are inconsistent with a desire to get well. They invite further decline in their health. This kind of person will not likely be healed, even if a whole church is praying for them (although, with God, all things are possible).

Sin

Jesus made it clear that not *all* disease can be traced back to sin. In a story told in John 9:1–3, Jesus was asked whose sin had caused a man to be blind, the man's sin or the sin of his parents. Jesus answered neither. Sin was *not* the cause. The man had been born blind "that the works of God might be displayed in him" (v. 3).

We considered (in the obedience chapter) that sickness can result from many causes that have nothing to do with personal sin: environmental toxins, chemicals added to food, bad genes, harmful pathogens, stress, and other causes that aren't our fault. They arise from the fallen world in which we live.

We also explored in that chapter that sometimes sickness is the result of sin. Psalm 107:17–18, for example, reveals: "Some were fools through their sinful ways, and because of their iniquities suffered affliction; they loathed any kind of food, and they drew near to the gates of death."

We should *not* condemn any sick person by thinking or saying they have sinned. During Job's season of suffering, his friends were convinced that Job's physical suffering could *only* be explained by sin. They told Job that he must have sinned and that God was punishing him. God set Job's friends straight.

We should never assume (like Job's friends) that someone else is sick, suffering, or dying because they have sinned. *Never*. We can only accurately judge our own selves. We are not to judge anyone else in this matter. We should only connect the dots between sin and sickness in another person *if* the person makes that connection and tells us so. It's not up to us to connect such dots.

Only God knows what's really going on in a person's heart:

> *... whatever sickness there is, whatever prayer, whatever plea is made by any man... each knowing the affliction of his own heart and stretching out his hands... then [Lord] hear in heaven... and forgive and act and render to each whose heart you know, according to all his ways (for you, you only, know the hearts of all the children of mankind)...*
>
> 1 Kings 8:37b–40

If we think that *possibly* sin has played a role in the ill health of another, we can pray for that person, that God will shine whatever light *He* wants to on whatever sin *might* exist. We should do this with a desire for the person's full healing (physical and spiritual), in a spirit of grace and compassion. We should *not* ask God to punish the person with ongoing sickness but instead plead for His mercy. We should *not* have the attitude that the person is getting what they deserve.

When we're sick, we can examine our own hearts, searching for sin. Thankfully, we can repent. Psalm 107:19–20 provides this example of what happened to people who had turned from their sin: "Then they cried to the Lord in their trouble, and he delivered them from their distress. He sent out his word and *healed* them, and delivered them from their destruction."

If you sense that sin thwarts prayers for your *own* healing, I encourage you to get right with God. Confess. Repent. Ask for His forgiveness, mercy, and grace. If we confess our sins, He is always faithful to cleanse and forgive us (1 John 1:9). *Then* ask for physical healing.

The Bible also counsels us to confess our sins to others. James 5:16a instructs: "…confess your sins to one another and pray for one another, that you may be healed." I'm not certain we have to confess our sins to other people in every circumstance. Each person has to prayerfully consider whether confession to another is a wise, appropriate route regarding any sin that might have harmed the other person.

A Hardened Heart

God told the prophet Isaiah to tell the Israelites they would not be healed because of their hardened hearts (Isaiah 6:9–10). God allows a person's heart to get hardened after a long period of disobedience.

On one occasion, Jesus told His disciples:

> … *You are permitted to understand the secrets of the Kingdom of Heaven, but others are not. To those who listen to my teaching, more understanding will be given… But for those who are not listening, even what little understanding they have will be taken away from them. That is why I use these parables, for they look, but they don't really see. They hear, but they don't really listen or understand. This fulfills the prophecy of Isaiah that says, "When you hear what I say, you will not understand. When you see what I do, you will not comprehend. For the hearts of these people are hardened, and their ears cannot hear, and they have closed their*

> *eyes—so their eyes cannot see, and their ears cannot hear, and*
> *their hearts cannot understand, and they cannot turn to me and*
> *let me heal them."*
> Matthew 13:11–15, NLT

Although it's less likely they'll do so, even those with hardened hearts can kneel at the foot of the cross, seeking forgiveness of their sins.

Fear and Other Destructive Thoughts and Emotions

Job stated, after a series of calamities beset him (including health woes), that what he had feared had come upon him (Job 3:25). We have discussed how much our thoughts and feelings can impact our health and the healing process, for better or worse. We have mentioned choosing faith instead of fear.

I love these words: "Strengthen the weak hands, and make firm the feeble knees. Say to those who have an anxious heart, 'Be strong; fear not!'" (Isaiah 35:3–4a). That prophet further recorded this message from God: "fear not, for I [the Lord] am with you; be not dismayed, for I am your God; I will strengthen you, I will help you, I will uphold you with my righteous right hand" (Isaiah 41:10).

We have talked about forgiveness. Before God restored Job, He asked Job to pray for the very friends who had condemned him (Job 42). Job did pray. He could only have sincerely done so if he had forgiven them. Forgiveness preceded restoration.

We have mentioned how various other unresolved issues, such as anger and resentment, can negatively impact our health and impede the healing process. Continue to examine all that is going on in your mind and heart.

Pride

Sometimes our pride holds us back from receiving healing. Perhaps we're embarrassed about a medical problem, so we don't tell our parents, spouse, friends, or doctor about it. Maybe we don't like to admit we're sick, weak, or unable to do something. We can be hesitant to reveal any imperfection. Pride can rob us of opportunities to receive prayer, biblical advice, pastoral care, medical help, practical support, and other assistance that could benefit us. We don't have to share *every* medical issue with others, but it's wise to share some of them, even if it's just with our doctor.

Counterfeit Healers

Some people have had bad experiences with counterfeit faith healers, which have made them cynical about further seeking healing from God. I recall one healing service I attended with a young man. The visiting evangelist called the young man forward and began praying for him, stating he believed that the man had leukemia. This person did not have that disease. His blood had been tested on numerous occasions during a recent hospitalization. If he had leukemia, it would have been detected. Years have passed and no leukemia has developed.

That one event wasn't enough to destroy my faith, or the faith of the young man, in God's healing power. We have both had good experiences (and biblical knowledge) to offset that one strange evening. Others have not been as fortunate.

Outright charlatans exist because they can profit from monetary offerings collected at itinerant healing services. We must be wary of snake oil salesmen. We must not, however, let past experiences with questionable "healers" rob us of a legitimate experience of God's healing power.

Viewing Suffering as a Lifelong "Cross" to Bear

Some people refer to their sickness or disability as the "cross" they bear. Jesus told His followers they would have to bear their own cross (see, for example, Mark 8:34). He made it clear that His followers would be persecuted, and perhaps even tortured or killed, just as He was. Suffering for *Him* and His Kingdom, however, is not the same as suffering because we're sick. Nowhere in the New Testament are we told that Jesus ever endured notable suffering from sickness. We can logically assume that when Jesus told His followers they would suffer, just as He suffered, He was not referring to suffering from physical disease. Not once in all of the gospel accounts do we read about Jesus telling a sick person to go home and endure their sickness.

The ennoblement of bodily suffering can be traced back to *pagan* thought in the centuries following Christ's death. The concept of Roman stoicism, for example, influenced the culture in which early believers lived.[63] By the fifth century, Christian leaders such as St. Gregory the Great were writing about the *virtue* of physical suffering and how much it benefitted the soul.[64] Suffering became a saintly activity. Physical suffering was sometimes self-inflicted.

Suffering *can* bless us in the ways I have listed in an earlier chapter, but seeing *some* value in a season of health-related suffering shouldn't replace the desire to be healed.

The healing revival of this past century rekindled belief in healing prayer in many denominations, yet many Christians will only call for their clergy, or the hospital chaplain, to either prepare them for death or to ask for help to endure suffering. Some don't ask for prayer for healing, believing that never-ending suffering is their assigned lot.

Aversion to Health and Wealth Teaching

Some pastors and authors unduly emphasize a health-and-wealth theology. This has caused many Christians, even some pastors, to steer clear of those topics. I agree that biblical teaching on health or wealth should not take centre stage. Our personal relationship with God must be of highest priority. Topics such as serving others, helping the poor, and leading others to Christ should receive due attention. Totally avoiding what the Bible says about physical needs, however, is just as extreme as putting the brightest spotlight on health and finances.

This book demonstrates that the Bible contains a large number of verses about health and healing. They may not be the most important verses in scripture, but their weighty existence is beyond dispute.

Paul said in Philippians 4:19 that God will supply *all* of our needs. In Philippians 4:6–7, he taught that we are not to worry about *anything* but to pray with thanksgiving about *everything*. Words such as "all," "anything," and "everything" are broad enough to cover our health and material needs, without making those needs paramount.

Clear the Way

I invite you to clear the way for God's healing power to come down. If you have recognized yourself in any of the above sections, or have been inwardly convicted at *any* point in this book, I encourage you to deal with whatever obstacle might be blocking God's healing power. If you're praying for someone else, then add to your prayers a request for God to help that person discover and remove any obstacles.

28

HEALED AT LAST

I hope this book has encouraged you. I hope you've grown in your understanding and use of the many points of access God has provided to His healing power. I am pausing to pray that your desired healing will come.

Often, healing is a combination of human effort and God's supernatural hand. Occasionally, God heals us without any human intervention. The best part about divine healing is that it happens without risks, complications, or negative side effects.

We cannot rely on any one method of healing or on only one point of access to God's healing power. What God did for someone else with a particular sickness might not be what He does for another person with that same plight. We cannot make assumptions about how and when God is going to act. We must simply put one foot in front of the next, obediently doing the many things He has told us to do, as best we can. If we continue on that path, I believe we will receive much healing over our lifetimes.

Seeking healing is not often easy. Within days of printing a draft manuscript of this book to obtain feedback from my first advance reader, I developed severe pain in my right abdomen. An ultrasound revealed that a large gallstone was blocking the neck of my gallbladder, with a second inch-wide gallstone just below it. Emergency surgery to remove my gallbladder occurred that same day. The surgeon (who specialized in such operations) told me that my gallbladder was the most enlarged, inflamed, and infected gallbladder she had ever seen. Some of the organ's tissue had become necrotic, posing the risk of internal gangrene developing and quickly spreading to other vital organs.

The surgery was longer and more complicated than usual. My enlarged gallbladder had to be dissected inside my abdomen, and a few large gallstones had to be crushed internally before their fragments could be removed through the small laparoscopic incisions. In the weeks post-surgery, I fought a painful abdominal infection that developed in the cavity where the gallbladder had been.

Some nights, both before and after the surgery, as I lay awake, I wondered how well I could put into practice what I had just finished writing about. Could I pray while feeling pain and fatigue? Could I meditate on various Bible verses and present them to God in petition? Could I exercise my faith? Could I trust Him? Could I praise Him? As I slowly recovered, I challenged myself: Could I thank Him for all that had gone right instead of focusing on what had gone wrong? I can now report that I did put this book (and its biblical principles) into practice as best I could. When my own vigour failed me, I relied on others to pray for me. We need not feel burdened by what God has instructed us to do. We just have to make *whatever* effort we can, however small. At times, we might only be able to whisper the name of Jesus. In those moments, that will be enough. I report with gratitude that I eventually recovered from both the surgery and the stubborn post-surgical infection.

Using each point of access to God's healing power becomes easier the more we put His instructions into practice. Activities such as praying, or remembering the promises and precedents in His Word, will become second nature when a health challenge arises.

I know of many more healing stories I could have told you. This book could be *much* longer. Dozens of people shared with me how God has healed them. I started writing about the stories closest to me (including my own) because I can vouch for their accuracy and I could supply details. I added in some other compelling stories I came across as I researched the topic of healing. I barely scratched the surface of my material before I ran out of space. It breaks my heart that I cannot honour every story I've been privileged to hear. I sincerely hope those stories are shared in other venues.

Many people have told me they have received substantial healing, or at least significant improvement, but they still want ongoing prayer for complete healing. So I will continue to pray for them. I hope that they continue to pray, too. I will also pray collectively for my readers, even if I don't have the opportunity to learn every name or need. God knows those details, and that's what matters above all.

The healing we receive in this life might not be perfect. We're imperfect people, surrounded by other imperfect people, living in an imperfect world. Our spiritual transformation isn't perfect. Our relationships aren't perfect. Why do we expect our health or our healing to be perfect? It may be that we have to accept that our health won't be perfect all the time. Only God is perfect. We won't be perfect, in our bodies or otherwise, until we meet Him in our eternal lives.

Perhaps God will improve our eyesight, but our vision may never become 20/20. When Jesus healed blind people while He was on earth, we don't know if their vision was restored to a perfect 20/20, but they were able to functionally see. I'm grateful that God has allowed us to live in an age in which glasses and contact lenses can improve our vision. We can thank God for such gifts.

By God's healing power, our mobility might significantly increase after an injury, but we might not be able to jump hurdles or run a marathon. Any measure of improvement is a great blessing. And, of course, we can keep asking for further healing.

Sometimes God provides a very great measure of healing. In the book of Job, Elihu talks about God restoring an adult's flesh to be like the skin of a child (Job 33:24–25). David talked in Psalm 103:5 about his youth being renewed. But we cannot always expect that we'll be perfectly restored to the physical condition we might have enjoyed as a younger person.

The healing we receive might not last as long as we'd like. Joy Davidman, the love of C. S. Lewis' life, was diagnosed with terminal bone cancer and prognosed with a brief time to live. Her pelvic bone had seriously and painfully deteriorated by the time of diagnosis. Lewis and others prayed for her. Remarkably, her pelvic bone somehow reconstructed itself. No medical explanation could account for this. She unexpectedly lived for a few more years, some of the happiest of her life. God provided a generous period of health before the cancer returned.

Let us celebrate *whatever* measure of healing we're granted for *as long* as it is granted. The miracle (of whatever God grants us) is *not* in our returning to yesterday's (or yesteryear's) superior state of physical being. The miracle lies in our ability to move forward, thankful for some measure of restored health for some further period of time. We should be thankful that we have lived another day, able to embrace whatever remains of this precious life we've been given. We can keep praying for a fuller measure of healing, but let's not count on perfect or permanent healing arriving in this world.

I trust and pray that God will heal you and me, over and over, of various ailments in our lifetimes here on earth. But if we live long enough to grow old, our body parts and systems will not all work as well as they once did. Moses lived to be 120, still strong and with good vision right to the end. We're told those two details, but we don't know the state of his hearing, digestive system, or blood pressure. In some terminal way, his body failed him at the end.

Unlike Moses, Isaac did *not* have good vision in his old age. (Jacob was able to trick his blind father into giving him the hands-on paternal blessing that should have been pronounced over his older brother, Esau, the firstborn son.) Ironically, by the end of his own life, Jacob's eyes "were dim with age, so that he could not see" (Genesis 48:10a).

King David lived to be old, passing the point of being able to take care of his own self. Bedridden, he needed the constant help of a young attendant (1 Kings 1:1–4, 15).

If you're advancing in years, maybe, like me, you have to wear glasses. Maybe, like me, you have to turn up the volume of the television. But we can still pray for a good measure of health, healing, strength, and energy.

At a certain point, we must all accept that our time on earth is drawing to an end, and we will be moving on to another, better place for the rest of eternity. We can take heart in our ultimate destiny.

I've heard the story of my husband's grandmother's death. Years before, I had the privilege of visiting her in Cairo. She had a faith in Christ that shone brightly in her eyes. I wish I'd been able to spend more time getting to know her better. When she was ninety-three years old, she was hospitalized with a stroke that left her blind, paralyzed on her left side, and unable to walk. She knew she likely had little time left to live. She spent some of her last days praying for her family and singing to the Lord, looking forward to being in His presence soon.

She prayed that she would be able to leave the hospital and die in her son's apartment, with family around her. That's what happened. She spent some final days with her loved ones at that apartment and then she went to be with her Lord.

The Lord promised that He has gone ahead of *all* believers to prepare a place for us. Jesus told His followers:

> *Let not your hearts be troubled. Believe in God; believe also in me.*
> *In my Father's house are many rooms. If it were not so, would I*
> *have told you that I go to prepare a place for you? And if I go and*
> *prepare a place for you, I will come again and will take you to*
> *myself, that where I am going you may be also.*
>
> John 14:1–3

In heaven, our resurrected bodies will never be sick or in agony. They will never bleed again. They will not waste away nor become weak and frail. In that coming day, our imperfect mortal bodies will be exchanged for immortal bodies that fully reflect their Creator's glory.

Listen to these words of Isaiah:

Strengthen the feeble hands, steady the knees that give way; say
to those with fearful hearts, 'Be strong, do not fear; your God
will come...' Then will the eyes of the blind be opened and the
ears of the deaf unstopped. Then will the lame leap like a deer,
and the mute tongue shout for joy... everlasting joy will crown
their heads. Gladness and joy will overtake them, and sorrow and
sighing will flee away.

Isaiah 35:3–6, 10bc, NIV

Some scholars say that Isaiah was prophesying in that passage about the future era when Jesus would minister to the sick and suffering here on earth. Many believe those verses *also* describe our future life in heaven because of the promise of "everlasting joy."

Revelation 21:4 paints this picture of heaven: "He [God] will wipe away every tear from their eyes, and death shall be no more, neither shall there be mourning, nor crying, nor pain anymore, for the former things have passed away."

If you are a fellow believer, I will see *you* there, in heaven. I imagine that you'll be strong, smiling, and radiant. You will be beautiful. Your eyes will sparkle, and your hair will shine. Your skin will be smooth. You will stand as straight as a sentry. You will walk, you will run, and you will laugh.

We will have resurrected and refashioned bodies that will be perfectly and permanently healthy. We shall together thank and praise God the Father, Jesus the risen Son, and the precious Holy Spirit, who so wonderfully befriended us, taught us, walked with us, offered us some measure of healing, and comforted us in the imperfect world we will have left behind. In our eternal home, we shall rejoice together that we have been *fully* healed at last.

Appendix A

A PRAYER TO ACCEPT CHRIST

If you would like to become a Christian, you can pray this prayer today:

Father God, I believe that You exist and that Jesus Christ is Your Son. I believe that Jesus died on the cross to pay the penalty for the sins of all humankind. I believe that He has risen and is now seated at Your right hand.

I confess that I'm a sinner. I choose to turn from known sins that come to mind and from all other sin. I ask You to please forgive *all* of my sins, on the basis of what Jesus did on the cross for *me*. Create in me a clean heart! Please remove my sins as far as the east is from the west. Please give me a fresh start in my life.

I give my life to You and ask You to be my Lord. I ask that You now dwell in me by Your Spirit, empowering me to live as I should. Thank You!

I pray in faith, in the name of Jesus Christ. Amen.

* * *

If you've prayed this prayer, you've made a new beginning in your life. The enemy of your soul will start to attack you with doubts and discouraging thoughts over the coming days. He will accuse you every time you slip up on your imperfect onward journey. Do not listen to him! Confess any new sins as they occur, turn from them, and ask God to forgive them, too. I encourage you to get a Bible and begin to read some verses every day, starting with the New Testament. Pray each day, talking to Father God in the name of Jesus. Ask to become better acquainted with the Holy Spirit who now lives within you. Find a Bible-believing church and start to make Christian friends. Grow in your ability to trust God and to obey Him. I will be praying for you.

Appendix B

———

A Short Prayer for Healing

Dear Father, I ask for the healing of [specify the need] for myself [or _____]. I ask for healing on the basis of Your love, kindness, compassion, mercy, and grace.

Please heal me [or _____] by: the power of Your Word, the power of my faith in Your Word, the power of prayer, the power of the cross, and the power of Your Spirit.

I offer to You my praise, love, gratitude, commitment, and trust.

Thank You for hearing my prayer. Thank You for what You will do in response, in Your timing. Thank You, in advance, for the measure of healing You will provide and the duration of life You will grant. I humbly, but boldly, ask for a great measure and a long duration. May my [his/her] healing bring You glory.

In Jesus' name I pray, Amen.

Appendix C

A LONGER PRAYER FOR YOUR HEALING

Dear Father, I come to You in the name of Your risen Son, Jesus Christ, who died on the cross for my sins so that I could have right standing with You. I confess my sins and seek Your forgiveness.

I praise and adore You, Lord God Almighty. I acknowledge Your unlimited power. Thank You for being my Creator, Sustainer, and Healer. Thank You for the gift of life and the measure of health, strength, and energy that You have already given me.

I now ask You to heal these parts of my body: _____. I ask for complete recovery from [sickness/injury/surgery/disability].

I appeal to Your love, kindness, compassion, mercy, and grace. Thank You for caring so much about me. I appeal to You on the basis of Your Word, especially the promises, precedents, and principles that pertain to healing. I believe Your Word is true and rest my faith upon it. You say, in Hebrews 11:6, that faith pleases You and that You reward faith. You say, in Matthew 17:20, that even if my faith is as tiny as a seed, it can move a mountain.

I lift up this prayer because You say, in James 5:16, that the prayer of a person in right standing with You is powerful and effective. John 14:13 tells me that I can ask for anything in the name of Jesus, and You will do it.

I trust You. You are trustworthy. I place my hope in You.

I value the cross and all that Jesus accomplished there for my whole being.

Please infuse me with more of the precious Holy Spirit. Please send Him to flow, like a river of living water, through every cell, system, and space in my body. Come, Holy Spirit, please come in greater measure. Please sustain my life. Please cause all pain to fade away. Please revive, renew, and restore my health. Please bring increased strength and energy, along with comfort and peace. Please cause all physical symptoms [e.g. bleeding, inflammation, infection, fever, fatigue] to subside and then disappear. Please wash away all disease, sickness, and every pathogen (including harmful bacteria and viruses). Please cause all physical dysfunction and disability to cease.

I now take up the power and authority You have granted me by Your Word, standing on verses such as Mark 16:17–18 and John 14:12. Jesus transferred all power and authority to heal to all who believe in Him, and that includes me. I pray aloud over my own body. I lay my hands on my own body. In cooperation with what the Spirit is doing within, I invite health, healing, strength, and energy into my body. I command all systems in my body to properly function as God created them to function.

In the name of Jesus, I command all sickness or disease to cease. I command all diseased or dysfunctional cells [including cancer cells] to shrivel up and die and disintegrate into nothingness. I command healthy cells to multiply. I banish sickness and disease from my body and command that they never return. I command all harmful pathogens to leave my body in orderly fashion. I declare that my body is the temple of the Spirit; therefore, sickness, disease, and disability have no rightful place in my body. Jesus has bought me with a great price.

I ask for wisdom regarding seeking medical help. If necessary, lead me to the right medical professionals. Guide me clearly, regarding: whether I should take medication(s), undergo surgery, or pursue any other medical therapies and procedures. Please also guide my doctor(s). Give them wisdom, knowledge, discernment, and skill. Help them to properly diagnose and treat me. Prompt them to order all necessary tests and to make all appropriate referrals to specialists. If You use medical means to heal me, may I remember to give You the ultimate credit.

Please send people to provide all of the practical support I need. I need help with: _____.

Please help me to take good care of my own body, as best I can. Help me to do *my* part in restoring and maintaining my health.

Please help me to be patient and persevering as I wait for healing to occur. Please help me to maintain faith, trust, and hope. Help me to get rid of [e.g. fear, worry, self-pity, discouragement] and other thoughts and feelings that are bothering me. Help me to keep on praying as long as it takes for my healing to come.

Please help me to endure whatever season of suffering I have to go through before I am healed. Let me discover great treasures in the darkness of my suffering. Help me to draw closer to You. You are the supreme treasure.

Please reveal to me any obstacles that are blocking my healing. Help me to take whatever steps I can to remove them.

May my healing bring You glory. You are worthy of all honour and glory.

Thank You for hearing my prayer. Thank You for what You will do in response, in Your timing. Thank You, in advance, for the measure of healing You will provide and the duration of life You will grant. I humbly, but boldly, ask for a great measure of healing and a long duration of life.

In Jesus' name I pray, Amen.

Appendix D

A LONGER PRAYER FOR THE
HEALING OF A LOVED ONE

[Please note that the italicized portions of this prayer apply only to believers. The rest of this prayer can be prayed over anyone who needs healing.]

Dear Father, I pray to You in the name of Your risen Son, Jesus Christ, who died on the cross so that I, a confessed sinner, can have right standing with You.

I praise and adore You, Lord God Almighty, acknowledging Your unlimited power. I thank You for creating and sustaining this person I am praying for: _____.

I ask for You to heal the following parts of [his/her] body: _____. I ask for [his/her] complete recovery from [sickness/injury/surgery/disability].

I appeal to Your love, kindness, compassion, mercy, and grace. Thank You for caring so much about [insert name].

I appeal to You on the basis of Your Word, especially the promises, precedents, and principles that pertain to healing. I believe Your Word is true and base my faith upon it. You say, in Hebrews 11:6, that faith pleases You and that You reward faith. You say, in Matthew 17:20, that even if my faith is as tiny as a seed, it can move a mountain.

Lord, I pray this prayer because You say, in James 5:16, that the prayer of a person in right standing with You is powerful and effective. Jesus said, in John 14:13, that I can ask for anything in His name, and You will do it.

I value the cross and all that Your Son, Jesus, accomplished there for [insert name].

Please infuse [insert name] with more of the Holy Spirit. Ask the Spirit to flow, like a river of living water, through every cell, system, and space of [his/her] body. Come, Holy Spirit, please come in greater measure. Please sustain their life. Please cause all pain to fade away. Please revive and restore [him/her]. Please bring increased strength and energy, along with comfort and peace. Please cause all symptoms to subside and then disappear. Please wash away all disease, sickness, and every pathogen (including harmful bacteria and viruses). Please cause all physical dysfunction and disability to cease.

I now take up the power and authority You have granted me by Your Word, standing on verses such as Mark 16:17–18 and John 14:12–13. Jesus transferred all power and authority to heal to *all* who believe in Him, and that includes me. I pray on behalf of [insert name]. With [his/her] permission, I lay my hands on their body. I speak health and healing into [his/her] body. I invite strength and energy to come. I command all systems in [his/her] body to properly function as God created them to function.

In the name of Jesus, I command all sickness, disease, and dysfunction to cease. I command all diseased or dysfunctional cells [including cancer cells] to shrivel up and die and disintegrate into nothingness. I command healthy cells to multiply. I banish sickness, disease, and dysfunction from the body of [insert name] and command that they never return. *I declare that [his/her] body is the temple of Your Spirit. I declare that sickness and disease have no rightful place in [his/her] body, because Jesus bought [him/her] with a great price.*

If necessary, lead [insert name] to the right medical professionals. Guide [him/her] clearly, regarding: whether or not to take medication(s), undergo surgery, or pursue other medical therapies and procedures. Please also guide [his/her] doctor(s). Give them wisdom, knowledge, discernment, and skill. Help them to properly diagnose and treat [insert their name]. Prompt them to order all necessary tests and to make all appropriate referrals to specialists. If You use medical means to heal [him/her], help them to give You the ultimate credit for their healing.

Please send people to provide all of the practical support [he/she] needs. [He/she] needs help with: _____.

Please help [him/her] to do their best to take good care of [his/her] body.

Please help [him/her] to be patient and persevering as [he/she] waits for healing to occur. *Please help [him/her] to maintain faith, trust, and hope.*

Please help [him/her] to endure whatever season of suffering [he/she] has to go through before healing comes. Help [him/her] to discover great treasures in the darkness of [his/her] suffering. Help [him/her] to draw closer to You. You are the supreme treasure.

Please reveal to [insert name] any obstacles that are blocking [his/her] healing. Help [him/her] to take whatever steps [he/she] can to remove them.

May the healing of [insert name] bring You glory.

Thank You for hearing my prayer and for what You will do in response, in Your timing. Thank You in advance for the measure of healing You will provide and the duration of life You will grant. I humbly and boldly ask for a great measure of healing and a long duration of life.

In Jesus' name I pray, Amen.

Contacting the Author

I love to hear from my readers. I value feedback. I would be very interested to hear what you have thought about this book. If you have any reactions, opinions, insights, or stories you wish to share, please contact me. Please also let me know about any prayer requests. I pray for my readers regularly. I can be reached at karenhenein@gmail.com. I am honoured that you have taken the time to read this book.

ENDNOTES

1   Dr. Richard Swenson, *More Than Meets the Eye: Fascinating Glimpses of God's Power and Design* (Colorado Springs, Colorado: NavPress, 2000), 17–20.

2   Ibid., 12, 23, 26–29, 36–40.

3   A. B. Simpson, *The Gospel of Healing* (Harrisburg, PA: Christian Publications, 1915), 45.

4   Josh McDowell, *Evidence That Demands a Verdict* (Nashville, TN: Thomas Nelson, 1979).

5   In biblical times, the term leprosy might have included other infectious skin diseases in addition to what we call leprosy today.

6   Agnes Sanford, *Sealed Orders* (Plainfield, NJ: Logos International, 1972), 259.

7   Allan Woods, "Guinness Records Guru on Extreme Old Age," *Toronto Star*, Jan. 19, 2016, A8; also see Guinness World Records at www.guinnessworldrecords.com, last accessed on November 3, 2018; also see pertinent statistics of the Gerontology Research Group, found at www.supercentenarian-research-foundation.org/TableE.aspx, last accessed on November 3, 2018. I have heard of one man in Asia who claims to be a little older than 120, but he does not have a birth certificate or other documentary evidence to prove it.

8   See, for example, an article by Jamie Ducharme, "You Asked: Do Religious People Live Longer?" published in the February 26, 2018 issue of *TIME* magazine. The article refers to various studies, including one co-authored by a Harvard professor, published in the prestigious *JAMA Internal Medicine* journal in 2016. That study found that women who attended more than one religious service per week had a 33% lower chance than secular women of dying during the sixteen years of the study. Data for that study was drawn from the 115,000-woman Nurse's Health Study. The *TIME* article also refers to the PLOS One study, co-authored by a professor at Vanderbilt University; that study found that regular worshippers were 55% less likely to die during the study's eighteen years of follow-up than those who did not attend religious services.

A ScienceDaily article, published in June of 2018, summarized a nationwide study of obituaries, undertaken by Ohio State University, which found that people with religious affiliation lived about four years longer than those with no religious affiliation.

See sciencedaily.com/releases/2018/06/180613163017.htm, last accessed on September 24, 2018. The study referred to is cited: Laura E. Wallace, Rebecca Anthony, Christian M. End, Baldwin M. Way, "Does Religion Stave Off the Grave? Religious Affiliation in One's Obituary and Longevity," *Social Psychological and Personality Science*, 2018 DOI: 10.1177/1948550618779820).

9   Leslie Montgomery, *The Faith of Condoleezza Rice* (Wheaton, IL: Crossway Books, 2007), 117, 120.

10   Justin Juozapavicius, "A Trailblazer of Televangelism," *Toronto Star*, December 16, 2009, A23.

11   Andrew Murray, *With Christ in the School of Prayer* (Springdale, PA: Whitaker House, 1981), 222.

12   Timothy Keller, *Prayer* (New York: Dutton Books, 2014), 111.

13   *ESV One Year Bible* (Wheaton, IL: Crossway, 2002), 30.

14   Brother Yun, *The Heavenly Man* (Grand Rapids, MI: Monarch Books, 2002) 23–25.

15   Ibid., 31–32.

16 Ibid., see, for example, 71, 75.

17 www.bibleengagmentstudy.ca.

18 Dodie Osteen, *Healed of Cancer* (Tulsa, Oklahoma: Harrison House Publishers, 1986).

19 A. B. Simpson, *The Gospel of Healing* (Chicago, IL: Moody Publishers, reprinted 2014).

20 My son's words are quoted from his typed notes of what he said at his baptism.

21 Catherine Marshall, *The Helper* (Grand Rapids, MI: Chosen Books, 2013), 176–177.

22 Justin Juozapavicius article.

23 Keller, 125.

24 J. I. Packer, *Knowing Christianity* (Wheaton, IL: Harold Shaw, 1995), 127.

25 Keller, 45, 62

26 Ibid., 97.

27 Francis MacNutt, *Healing* (Notre Dame, IN: Ava Maria Press, 1999 revised edition), 7.

28 Ibid., 34–35.

29 This website was last accessed on November 10, 2018.

30 www.stormieomartian.com (last accessed on March 14, 2018); click on "prayer community."

31 MacNutt, *Healing*, 19; see further references footnoted on 19; I have not personally read every study referred to.

32 See, for example, these articles: K. A. Matthews, K. Raikkonen, K. Sutton-Tyrrell, and L. H. Kuller, "Optimistic Attitudes Protect Against Progression of Carotid Atherosclerosis in Healthy Middle-aged Women," *Psychosomatic Medicine* 66 (2004), 640-644; D. D. Danner, D. A. Snowden, and W. V. Friesen, "Positive Emotions in Early Life and Longevity; Findings from the Nun Study," *Journal of Personality and Social Psychology* 80 (2001), 804-813.

33 Dr. Mario Beauregard and Denyse O'Leary, *The Spiritual Brain: A Neuroscientist's Case for the Existence of the Soul* (New York: Harper Collins, 2007), 141, 144.

34 Francis MacNutt, *The Healing Reawakening*, (Grand Rapids, MI: Chosen Books, 2005), 41.

35 Murray, 181.

36 Brother Andrew, *Light Force* (Grand Rapids, MI: Fleming H. Revell, 2004), see, for example, 124.

37 F. F. Bosworth, *Christ the Healer* (Grand Rapids, MI: Fleming H. Revell, 1973), 61.

38 Dr. Swenson, 26.

39 John W. Kennedy, "The Crusader," *Christianity Today*, November 2013.

40 MacNutt, *Healing*, 46–47; MacNutt, *The Healing Reawakening*, especially 69, 87, 131, 140–141, 146–151, 162–163, 172–183.

41 Ibid., 13.

42 Brian Stiller, "Argentina: An Epic Faith," *Dispatches from the Global Village*, June 2016.

43 Brother Andrew, *For the Love of My Brothers* (Minneapolis: Bethany House, 1998), 52–53.

44 MacNutt, *Healing*, 7.

45 Ibid., 131.

46 Unknown author, "Faith Healing Death Draws Jail Time," *Christianity Today*, December 2009.

47 Kim Kuo, "Giving Our Final Days to God," *Christianity Today*, September 2015.

48 Steve Buist, "Patient, Heal Thyself," *Toronto Star*, February 27, 2016, IN6.

49 Jennifer Yang, "UN Debates 'Apocalyptic' Threat of Superbugs," *Toronto Star*, Sept. 21, 2016, A10.

50 Brother Andrew, *God's Smuggler* (Grand Rapids, MI: Chosen, 2015 expanded edition).

51 Brother Andrew, *For the Love of My Brothers*, 57–62.

52 J. K. Kiecolt-Glaser, I. McGuire, T. F. Robles, and R. Glaser, "Emotions, Morbidity, and Mortality: New Perspectives from Psychoneuroimmunology," *Annual Review of Psychology* 53 (2002), 83–107; B. L. Fredrickson, "What Good Are Positive Emotions?"

Review of General Psychology 2 (1998), 300–319; B. L. Fredrickson and R. W. Levenson, "Positive Emotions Speed Recovery from the Cardiovascular Sequelae of Negative Emotions," *Cognition and Emotion* 12 (1998), 191–220; M. M. Herrald and J. Tomaka, "Pattern of Emotion-Specific Appraisal, Coping, and Cardiovascular Reactivity During an Ongoing Emotional Episode," *Journal of Personality and Social Psychology* 83 (2002), 434–450; Everson, et al, "Hostility and Increased Risk of Mortality and Acute Myocardial Infarction: The Mediating Role of Behavioral Risk Factors," *American Journal of Epidemiology* 146, no. 2 (1997), 142–152; R. C. Kneip, A. M. Delamater, T. Ismond, C. Milford, L. Salvia, and D. Schwartz, "Self and Spouse Ratings of Anger and Hostility as Predictors of Coronary Heart Disease," *Health Psychology* 12 (1993), 301–307; L. D. Kubzansky, I. Kawachi, A. Spiro III, S. T. Weiss, P. S. Vokonas, and D. Sparrow. "Is Worrying Bad for Your Heart? A Prospective Study of Worry and Heart Disease in the Normative Aging Study," *Circulation* 95 (1997), 818–824.

53   Karen Henein, *Bent Out of Shape* (Canada: Word Alive Press, 2008).

54   MacNutt, *Healing*, 8–11.

55   Ibid., 25.

56   Brother Andrew, *God's Smuggler*, 30–35, 57–58.

57   Kuo article.

58   Stormie Omartian, *Out of Darkness* (Oregon: Harvest House, 2015).

59   Omartian.

60   Kay Warren, *Choose Joy* (Grand Rapids, MI: Revell, 2012).

61   Billy Graham, *Storm Warning* (Nashville, TN: Thomas Nelson, 1995 new edition).

62   Ibid., 36.

63   MacNutt, *Healing*, 49.

64   Ibid., 51.

ALSO FROM KAREN HENEIN

These three non-fiction books each contain hundreds of verses, laying a strong biblical foundation for the topics they discuss. The books relate stories from the lives of the author, her family and friends, and well-known Christians, past and present, that illustrate practical application of key principles.

Counsel of the Most High: Receiving God's Guidance for Life's Decisions
ISBN # 9781894928991
Word Alive Press, 2007

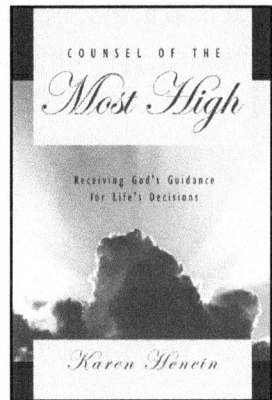

This book explores how we can wisely make the "big" decisions in our lives while also receiving God's guidance for more minor, everyday choices. Readers can learn how to discern God's plans and purposes for their lives. A single footstep may seem insignificant but over time, our footsteps take us in one direction or another. Our daily footsteps matter!

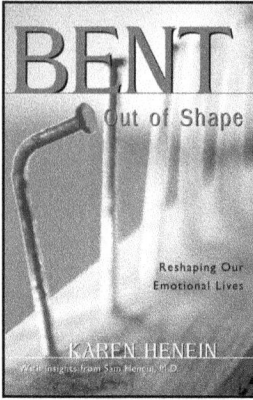

Bent Out of Shape:
Reshaping Our Emotional Lives
ISBN # 9781897373446
Word Alive Press, 2008

This book discusses how to move from distressing feelings (such as anger, resentment, fear, worry, discouragement, and depression) to positive mental and emotional states such as forgiveness, love, peace, faith, hope, and joy. It contains insights from Christian medical doctors (including her husband), psychologists, psychiatrists, and pastors.

Seeking the Truth About Money
ISBN # 9781770692879
Word Alive Press, 2011

This book provides a comprehensive and balanced view on how Christians can integrate wise inner attitudes toward money with practical activities such as acquiring, saving, investing, spending, and giving money.

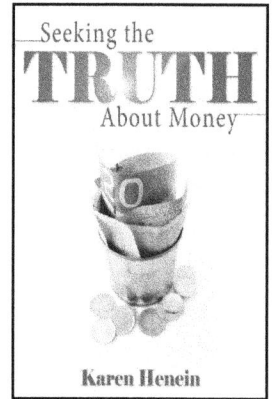

www.ingramcontent.com/pod-product-compliance
Lightning Source LLC
Chambersburg PA
CBHW060002100426
42740CB00010B/1375